BENEDICT MEDICINE

A Catholic Response to Rescue the Profession's Healing Mission

James O. Breen

BENEDICT MEDICINE LLC
Fort Myers, Florida

Cover image: Detail of "Christ Healing the Sick," by Heinrich Hofmann, 1893.

Graphic design, editorial, and other book packaging services provided by FastEditing LLC, Jeanette Fast Redmond, Owner, www.fastediting.biz.

ISBN-13 (print): 979-8-218-75542-3
ISBN-13 (ebook): 979-8-218-75555-3

First printing, September 2025

Contents

II. A Manual for Reclaiming the *Telos* of Medicine

Introduction

"Tradition refuses to submit to the small and arrogant oligarchy of those who merely happen to be walking about."

—G. K. Chesterton[1]

What is the purpose of medicine? What is the call that countless doctors, nurses, and other medical personnel have answered when they dedicated themselves to minister to the sick? From where did this calling come, and what role has it played in the development of Western civilization and our understanding about what it means to be human? Finally, what has caused the medical profession in the West to lapse so profoundly from its original purpose of bringing about healing and promoting authentic human flourishing?

That our healthcare system suffers from a chronic and deeply debilitating illness comes as no revelation to the average American. Our ailing medical system—here, the patient—is chronically ill and has not really been well for a long time. The problem goes far beyond the material effects of the malady, which include increasing wait times for decreased access to care; impersonal, homogeneous, corporate bureaucratic structures; increasing insurance and out-of-pocket costs for more restricted care; and the depersonalization of care, leading to patient mistrust and caregiver alienation. These are merely symptoms of the affliction plaguing the US healthcare system. Beyond mere organizational mismanagement, a deep spiritual malaise lies at the root of the healthcare enterprise. That the bureaucracy has failed to satisfy people's deeper needs for humanizing medical care only highlights how the nation's healthcare apparatus neglects medicine's deeper purpose.

Rather than reflecting the *telos*—the ultimate end, or right purpose—of medicine, the commentariat and political leaders consider healthcare in terms beneficial to their aims. On its surface, the financial and organizational arrangement upon which we depend for medical care has been a hot-button issue at the center of political wrangling for decades, causing deep divisions among generations of Americans. In popular debates, the crux of the healthcare divide relies on a false premise: that the solution to the US healthcare debacle can be found through either (1) greater

[1] G. K. Chesterton, *Orthodoxy* (Dodd, Mead & Company, 1908; Image Classics, 2001), 45.

expansion of the government safety net or (2) increased market freedom within the health sector. Thus, the perceived root of America's healthcare woes can be summarized by the following question: Should healthcare be treated as a basic right that is guaranteed and provided by government, or should access to medical services instead be directed by the invisible hand of the market? Americans have long debated the proper role of government in the way medical professionals and other healthcare stakeholders are regulated and incentivized to behave. Sadly, today's US healthcare system combines the most pernicious aspects of both government control and free-market healthcare: suffocating state regulation and the attendant rising costs, coupled with the depersonalizing commoditization of big-business capitalism.

By limiting itself solely to the financial structure of medical care, the prevailing structure debases the motivations of healthcare workers by considering us in one-dimensional economic terms, rather than acknowledging the intangible human forces that compel many of us to pursue a medical vocation. Hence, political liberals and progressives agitate for expanding government to provide publicly sponsored healthcare to a wider swath of Americans. At the same time, fiscal conservatives as well as libertarians support reducing the role of government in healthcare services, based largely on the idea that government subsidizing of healthcare markets creates a fiscal dependency on government and distorts the prices of healthcare-related goods and services. Oscillating across numerous election cycles, the pendulum has tended to swing ever more leftward since the creation of Medicare and Medicaid in the mid-1960s. This swing has led to an increased role of federal and state governments in healthcare, as highlighted in recent decades by the passage of the 2010 Patient Protection and Affordable Care Act (ACA) and continued efforts on the part of the political left to incentivize greater federal expansion of the Medicaid rolls in states that have resisted offers of federal subsidies.

The Effect of Partisan Politics

As with many controversial issues affecting civic life, most Americans don their partisan political hats when considering the healthcare dilemma. In a country and culture that have thoroughly privatized any notion of belief or existential meaning, political leanings offer a comfortable and safe—if somewhat superficial—way to approach publicly a topic of such crucial importance to the actual health of our citizenry and the fiscal health of our country. The perennial national debate around healthcare—perpetuated by political parties, medical societies, pharmaceutical companies, insurance lobbies, and other interest groups—all paint the conflict in strictly economic and political terms. Ironically, far from seeking compromise and a peaceful resolution, these stakeholders all have much to gain by perpetuating the dispute. In the perennial ebb and flow of election cycles, the major political parties channel the vitriol created by national healthcare politics in order to buttress voter support from sympathizers. Medical societies like the American Medical Association (AMA) alert physician-constituents and the public to share how they are hard at work lobbying on behalf of healthcare equity and the profession—as they plaintively ask for doctors' support at the same time. Political lobbies such as the American Association of Retired People and other special interest groups sound alarms about threats to Medicare and other legislative battles with implications for their constituencies. Sadly, for all the distractions created by these partisans, we do not seem to be any closer to consensus—or to a shared vision of what a humanized healthcare system looks like.

Western Medical Tradition and Christianity

For the 63% of Americans who identify as Christian, a question arises.[2] Rather than considering the issue along the partisan divide, how might we interpret the direction of our national healthcare infrastructure as followers of Christ, specifically informed by the principles of Catholic social teaching?[3] Most importantly, how do we define the true ends—the *telos*—of medicine, and properly align practice with purpose?

In this book, I assert that we must do exactly that. But first, the medical tradition of Hippocrates has been a hallmark of Western civilization since at least the third century BC, grounding the physician's approach to clinical care today and the modern development of bioethics. From the ancient Greek healer's solemn invocation of spiritual help in practicing the medical craft, to the foundational axiom "*primum non nocere*" (first do no harm—attributed to Hippocrates, though not mentioned specifically in his oath), Western medicine has always derived a great deal of authority from appealing to the transcendent purpose behind the physician's work.

Building on the pre-Christian Greek belief that the practice of medicine implies a hallowed oath, the Judeo-Christian concept of *imago Dei* imparted to the medical practitioner the sacred belief that every human being is endowed with immeasurable dignity because he or she is created

---

2 Pew Research Center, "After Years of Decline, the Christian Share of the U.S. Population Stabilizes," February 14, 2025, https://www.pewresearch.org/religion/2025/02/26/decline-of-christianity-in-the-us-has-slowed-may-have-leveled-off/pr_2025-02-26_religious-landscape-study_0-01/.

3 Pew Research Center, "How U.S. Religious Composition Has Changed in Recent Decades," September 13, 2022, https://www.pewresearch.org/religion/2022/09/13/how-u-s-religious-composition-has-changed-in-recent-decades/.

in the image and likeness of God. As Jesus' divine commandment suggests, the *imago Dei* requires the medical practitioner to honor the duty to safeguard all human life in practicing the medical profession. Deriving from this concept, the Christian concept of *agape* love—that is, unconditional in nature, mirroring God's love for humanity—further transformed medical practice into a selfless act of Christian charity, just as our Lord described in the parable of the Good Samaritan (see Luke 10:29–37).

Today, the transcendent values that formed the backbone of Western society and medical tradition alike are being actively and systematically negated at an accelerated pace. This development is one of many negative downstream effects caused by unmooring the broader culture from any transcendent belief system. Rather than being defined by a uniting supernatural worldview, today's prevailing secular culture is characterized by a deep and abiding cynicism arising from a loss of faith—faith in God, in the goodwill of our fellow citizens, and in the institutions once heralded as signs of national exceptionalism. The concepts of our nation's Declaration of Independence—"that all men are created equal, that they are endowed by their Creator with certain unalienable Rights, that among these are Life, Liberty and the pursuit of Happiness"—have been deemed incompatible with the new contemporary creed. Mainstream pundits label as "extremist" the idea that our rights are endowed by the Almighty.[4] The God of *imago Dei* has been subverted by a focus on group identity that overrides the Christian focus on the commonalities among all people as made in God's likeness and image. Contemptuous ideas of relativism have undermined the common intellectual heritage that binds all Americans irrespective of when or how they arrived on these shores.

Symptoms of Desperation

Tragically, evidence of widespread desperation is not hard to find. At a time when Western societies enjoy the highest degree of material prosperity and comfort ever known, diagnoses of depression and anxiety are increasing at a record pace. A 2023 Gallup survey reported the highest-ever percentage of American adults who have ever been diagnosed with depression: 29%, up from 19.6% in 2015. Similarly, the incidence of depression in 2023 was also the highest ever among adults at 18%,

---

[4] See Heidi Przybyla, interview on MSNBC, February 23, 2024, posted by Tim Hains, "Heidi Przybyla: Extremist Conservative Christian Nationalists Believe Your Rights Come from God, not Government," RealClearPolitics, February 23, 2024, https://www.realclearpolitics.com/video/2024/02/23/heidi_przybyla_extremist_conservative_christian_nationalists_believe_your_rights_come_from_god_not_government.html.

compared to just 10% eight years earlier.[5] According to the National Center for Health Statistics (NCHS), suicide—another marker of despair—has become the second-leading cause of death among American young people between the ages of 10 and 24 between 2011 and 2021, while also increasing 63% among 20- to 24-year-olds from 2001 to 2021.[6] The NCHS also reported in 2023 that addiction rates and overdose-related deaths are skyrocketing—despite (or perhaps abetted by) widespread educational campaigns and "harm reduction" strategies, such as needle exchange programs and medically supervised drug consumption sites, seeking to stem the tide.[7]

A pervasive cultural nonconformity with objective truths appears to parallel the rise in the symptoms of despair. As an example, the number of young people who dispute their genetic and biological status as male or female is evident in the exponential rise in self-identified "nonbinary" or "transgender" young adults, as reported by Gallup in 2024—up to 2.8% among members of Generation Z (birth years 1997–2012). Dissent from societal sexual norms is also evidenced in the dramatic increase of LBGTQ+ identification, with a nearly tenfold increase among the young—from 2.3% of baby boomers (born 1946–64) to 22.3% of Generation Z.[8] Far from reinforcing self-evident and long-held truths about human sexuality, many Western societies have sought to celebrate and encourage the concept of the sexually "fluid" individual.

The thirty-thousand-foot view suggests that increasing opulence coincides with societal markers of hopelessness and rejection of cultural anchors. Increased material wealth also appears to be inversely related to adherence to religious belief and faith in God. In 2023 the Pew Research Center reported that 28% of American adults do not hold a religious affiliation.[9] In 2007, according to Pew, the percentage of Americans self-described as "nones" was a mere 17%—but that itself was up from less

---

5 Dan Witters, "U.S. Depression Rates Reach New Highs," Gallup, May 17, 2023, https://news.gallup.com/poll/505745/depression-rates-reach-new-highs.aspx.

6 Sally C. Curtin and Matthew F. Garnett, *Suicide and Homicide Death Rates Among Youth and Young Adults Aged 10–24: United States, 2001–2021* (National Center for Health Statistics [NCHS] Data Brief No. 471, June 2023), https://www.cdc.gov/nchs/data/databriefs/db471.pdf.

7 Merianne R. Spencer, Matthew F. Garnett, and Arialdi M. Miniño, *Drug Overdose Deaths in the United States, 2002–2022* (NCHS Data Brief No. 491, March 2024), https://www.cdc.gov/nchs/data/databriefs/db491.pdf.

8 Jeffrey M. Jones, "LGBTQ+ Identification in U.S. Now at 7.6%," Gallup, March 13, 2024, https://news.gallup.com/poll/611864/lgbtq-identification.aspx.

9 Pew Research Center, "Religious 'Nones' in America: Who They Are and What They Believe," January 24, 2024, https://www.pewresearch.org/religion/2024/01/24/religious-nones-in-america-who-they-are-and-what-they-believe/.

than 10% in the 1980s, as reported by Gallup.[10] The generational aspect of the increase in the religiously unaffiliated is evident: while 29% of US adults under age 30 identify as "nones," only 13% of those 65 years and older fall into that category.[11] And while correlation does not imply causation, the implications for a continued trend toward increasing hopelessness and detachment from transcendent belief are ominous.

Closely aligned with other measures of hopelessness, the phenomenon of burnout across a wide range of work disciplines (including, prominently, in medicine) has received increased attention in recent years. Social science characterizes burnout as including emotional exhaustion, decreased efficacy, and negative perceptions of oneself.[12] Though researchers have taken an intense interest in the causes and effects of burnout, one critical contributing factor is the loss of a sense of meaning and purpose. Particularly for healthcare workers animated by faith, severing the connection between public work and private beliefs contributes to a deep sense of loss. In a professional environment—where healthcare professionals of faith are compelled to present sharp distinctions between outward secular personae at odds with an inner spiritual life—this disconnect leads to a quiet privatization of belief that erodes a professional sense of purpose. The result of this cognitive and spiritual dissonance between public and private faces is that those of us who entered our medical careers animated by a vibrant faith feel forced to make compromises in order to get along professionally. In essence, the secular medical culture compels us to conduct our public, professional lives in ways that deny God.

While much has been written about the effects of secularization on society at large, less attention has been given to the neutralization of faith and its influence on the medical profession. Recognizing how secularized US medicine is inimical to its Christian inheritance can help Christian medical professionals and nonclinicians alike to recognize the pernicious effects of this accelerating secularization. For the layperson of faith, distinguishing between the historical transcendence of medical ethics and the contemporary ethos of secular medicine helps one decide how to engage with the healthcare system while maintaining a properly ordered Christian life. For medical professionals, an appreciation of these competing worldviews allows us to understand the cause of malaise and thus to respond in ways that bear witness to the truth and

---

[10] Frank Newport, "Slowdown in the Rise of Religious Nones," Gallup, December 9, 2022, https://news.gallup.com/opinion/polling-matters/406544/slowdown-rise-religious-nones.aspx.

[11] Pew Research Center, "Religious 'Nones' in America."

[12] See "What Is Burnout?" Cleveland Clinic, February 1, 2022, https://health.clevelandclinic.org/signs-of-burnout#What%20Is%20Burnout.

rehabilitate our sense of purpose—in essence, to recover medicine's *telos* in our day-to-day practice of medicine.

Catholic Social Teaching and Medicine

Fortunately, the Catholic Church has given us the great gift of a detailed map and accurate compass in our quest to rediscover the transcendental meaning of medicine. The principles of Catholic social teaching are based on the teachings of our Lord found in Scripture and Tradition and were first articulated in modern times by Pope Leo XIII in his 1891 encyclical *Rerum novarum*. The principles of Catholic social teaching orient our thoughts and direct our actions in an authentically Christian way with regard to social issues.[13] In *Rerum novarum*, Leo XIII addressed the dignity of workers and their rights to the fruits of their labor, in opposition to the rising tides of both socialism and unregulated capitalism of his time. In the ensuing decades, a multitude of papal encyclicals cast greater light on various aspects of the application of Catholic social doctrine. Pope St. John Paul II's 1981 encyclical *Laborem exercens* addressed the rights of workers and the dignity of work, while his 1995 encyclical *Evangelium vitae* vigorously asserted the inherent dignity of every human life from conception to natural death.[14] Pope Benedict XVI, in his 2009 encyclical *Caritas in veritate*, addressed the issue of poverty in a globalizing world, asserting that the aftereffects of a globalism oriented solely toward profit can only be addressed by speaking truth motivated by charitable love.[15] Far from being an exhaustive treatise, this paragraph offers a glimpse into the historical understanding of the Church's teaching on social issues, points toward primary sources for further reading, and suggests how the Church's teaching should inform our approach to contemporary societal topics.

In its treatment of Catholic social teaching, the United States Conference of Catholic Bishops organizes its teaching around seven principles

---

[13] Leo XIII, Encyclical *Rerum novarum* (*On Capital and Labor*), May 15, 1891, https://www.vatican.va/content/leo-xiii/en/encyclicals/documents/hf_l-xiii_enc_15051891_rerum-novarum.html.

[14] John Paul II, Encyclical *Laborem exercens* (*On Human Work*), September 14, 1981, https://www.vatican.va/content/john-paul-ii/en/encyclicals/documents/hf_jp-ii_enc_14091981_laborem-exercens.html; John Paul II, Encyclical *Evangelium vitae* (*On the Value and Inviolability of Human Life*), March 25, 1995, https://www.vatican.va/content/john-paul-ii/en/encyclicals/documents/hf_jp-ii_enc_25031995_evangelium-vitae.html.

[15] Benedict XVI, Encyclical *Caritas in veritate* (*On Integral Human Development in Charity and Truth*), June 29, 2009, https://www.vatican.va/content/benedict-xvi/en/encyclicals/documents/hf_ben-xvi_enc_20090629_caritas-in-veritate.html.

of this vast and far-reaching subject. To streamline such an expansive topic, I distill the elements of Catholic social teaching into four overarching principles: (1) dignity of the human person, (2) solidarity, (3) subsidiarity, and (4) effective stewardship of resources. That is, committed Christians deepen their commitment to Jesus Christ as the transcendent Truth and to one another by how we address social concerns in medicine: first, by understanding the meaning and importance of the inherent dignity of the human person as made in the image and likeness of God; second, through the call to work in solidarity for the common good of all, including the weak and vulnerable; third, by encouraging decision making to take place at the lowest level of community possible, also known as the principle of subsidiarity; and finally, by honoring God's gifts through effective stewardship of resources.

Further examination of these principles makes us keenly aware of the many ways the prevailing healthcare system routinely subverts Christian ethics, thereby distancing medical practice from its right-ordered purpose. Disquietingly, this awareness of the mismatch between the current secular medical culture and Christian principles challenges us to recognize the implications of this ongoing incompatibility—both for ourselves as individual patients and professionals, and for the integrity of society more broadly. No longer can we be complacent in the muddled middle. The unease that comes with this increased awareness compels the Christian to action.

While a solid understanding of Catholic social teaching is critical to formulate an effective response to secularism's assault on medical practice, it is not sufficient. For believing Christians, a robust answer necessarily depends on an outpouring of grace from the Holy Spirit to allow radical hope to take hold of our minds and hearts. A deep prayer life, continual discernment (asking God to reveal his plan for our lives), and cultivation of a sacramentally centered life are all essential parts of this process.

About This Book

The book you are holding has been divided into two parts, each further subdivided into chapters.

Part One presents a brief introduction of Western medicine's Judeo-Christian inheritance and defines terms to aid later exploration of Catholic social teaching principles and the ways in which the prevailing secular medical culture violates them. Chapter 1 provides this overview of how Christian belief birthed the foundational precepts of Western medicine and of how the West's current loss of transcendent belief has eroded medicine's legitimacy. Then chapter 2 examines, in broad strokes, the basic principles of Catholic social teaching as a Christian framework for addressing social issues in medical care.

Informed by this understanding of Catholic social teaching, chapter 3 analyzes the contemporary US healthcare system according to Catholic social teaching principles as a means of bringing the stark contrasts into clearer focus. My observations about the relationship between Catholic social teaching and secular healthcare form the framework for considering an authentically Catholic form of primary medical care. "Benedict Medicine"—the term promoted by the title of this book—refers to the outcome of this analysis, namely, a set of characteristics of primary care oriented toward authentic human flourishing and the alleviation of suffering, as directed by Catholic social teaching.

In chapter 4, which concludes Part One, I explore language as the medium by which we develop habits of thought when considering the topics of medicine and ethics. Many words and terms that previously were commonly understood—for example, words referring to virtues, vices, and human sexuality—have had their meanings altered in the current lexicon. To name just a few examples, in today's secular morality, pride is a virtue and chastity a pitiable deprivation. The concept of gender as something distinct from sex is promoted as self-intuitive and beyond question. In the same way contemporary language erases distinctions between the sexes, it also downplays differences among the roles and functions of different medical professionals (as with the term "healthcare provider," to cite one example). Unknowing acceptance of newly minted definitions, and the adoption of this newfangled vocabulary, creates false habits of mind and unconsciously modifies the way we think about these topics.

Part Two of the book then offers a practical guide to implementing Benedict Medicine. It serves as a manual for reclaiming medicine's purpose as an expression of Christian charity and the corporal works of mercy. Chapter 5 outlines the pillars of the Benedict Medicine project, beginning with the premise that for Christians, reimagining medical practice as a faith-inspired action is not intended to be a private activity. Such reimagining requires clinicians and nonclinicians alike to consider our role in building up Christian communities, which themselves serve as fortresses to protect us from danger and as leaven to grow and sustain the faith of servant and served alike. This reenvisioned approach to medical care demands that we profess an unapologetic adherence to the truth by living an integrated life in which our private revelations are concordant with our public actions. The natural outcome of developing an outwardly Catholic approach to medical care is the formation of tangible witness in the world.

A contemporary example of a similar phenomenon comes from the world of K-12 education: namely, the growth of the Catholic classical education movement, through which committed families come together to establish schools that nurture their children both academically and spiritually. The historical blueprint for such an approach to Christian renewal is nowhere better illustrated than through the life of St. Benedict of Nursia, founder of Western monasticism, whose flight to a cave in Subiaco, Italy, in the sixth century led to the preservation of Christianity during a time of great societal corruption. Indeed, the life of St. Benedict was the example that Rod Dreher gave in his book *The Benedict Option* about the need for the faithful to form community to survive the corruption of our current times.[16] I owe no small debt to Dreher for prompting me to consider how his Benedict option might apply to modern medicine.

The later chapters of part two apply the principles of Catholic social teaching to medicine as a means to map out a practical model of contemporary Catholic witness in the medical culture. Examples of existing approaches that embody elements of Catholic social teaching and enliven the Catholic creative imagination provide substance to the frame described in chapter 5, illustrating in a medical context the concept of human dignity, the twin principles of solidarity and subsidiarity, and pragmatic examples of prudential stewardship.

In chapter 6, I explain why primary care is a natural starting point for reconstituting a Catholic medical response to the afflictions affecting the prevailing healthcare system. In my role as a faculty physician who has taught medical students and residents for many years, I have repeatedly reminded trainees that the primary care physician is the specialist in the "undifferentiated complaint." He or she must interpret the patient's description of the problem (detailed in the medical history), combine it with observations from the physical exam, and add information derived from targeted diagnostic testing to arrive at a diagnosis. Most people, when they encounter a new symptom or problem, begin their medical sojourn in the exam room of their primary care physician. Because primary care is open to all people, irrespective of age or sex, in the communities where they live and work; because it offers the potential to identify medical conditions earlier in their course; and because it requires the least material resources of any sector within the healthcare system—for all these reasons, primary care is the logical linchpin for any effort to renew medical practice according to the pillars of Benedict Medicine.

This book is written with both medical professionals and laypeople in mind, because healthcare touches every person's life at some point. Because I am writing as a Catholic primary care physician, this book necessarily approaches the subject from a distinctively Catholic point of view. Nevertheless, it is my hope that the observations in this book will also interest non-Catholic Christians who share in the hope for a revitalization of Western medical practice that reflects its Christian

---

[16] See Rod Dreher, *The Benedict Option* (Sentinel Press, 2017).

foundations. Furthermore, for Christians, the work of building up the Kingdom is the Great Commission to which all the baptized are called. Although many of the observations seem to focus on the perspective of medical professionals, nonclinical readers will find the insights useful as they consider more deeply their own encounters with the healthcare system and the choices that flow from those interactions. Ultimately, doctors' professional vocations have no meaning if they are not serving patients, and patients must place their trust in doctors' expertise and recommendations when they find themselves at their most vulnerable. The task of constructing an approach to medical care that honors its *telos*, in service of the truth and informed by the principles of Catholic social teaching, is the essence of Benedict Medicine. At its heart, the interconnectedness of clinicians with those they serve exemplifies how we are called to serve out the commission that Christ ordained.

Part I

The Assault on the Purpose of Medicine

CHAPTER 1

Western Medicine and Its Roots in the Church

"Many are the sick people in the hospital of this present age. The same medicine does not fit them all, nor is the same diet right for all. The physician (Christ) assigns the medicines and diet appropriate for each patient."

—St. Neilos of Ancyra[1]

The date is May 8, 1642. Upon the shores of the island of Montreal, a young French nurse and laywoman named Jeanne Mance arrives with her party of missionaries to establish a community of Christian charity in service to the colonists of what was then New France and to the land's Indigenous inhabitants. Erected at the base of Mount Royal, the new town of Ville-Marie (now a borough of Montreal) is distinctive because of its *hôtel-Dieu*, or "God shelter," founded to bring healing to the sick and to alleviate the suffering of all who came for care. This early new-world hospital serves as the origin of the North American ministry of the Religious Hospitallers of St. Joseph, founded by Mance.[2]

The impact of these courageous souls, who braved the ocean and the primitive conditions in New France to minister to the sick, cannot be overstated. With faith and determination, the missionary group who settled Montreal and its hôtel-Dieu—including Mance and patron Paul De Chomedey de Maisonneuve—overcame long, frigid winters, shortages of material supplies, and the arrows of the local Iroquois as they set about establishing a Christian outpost in the wilderness. For three hundred years, the Religious Hospitallers of St. Joseph were instrumental in founding an additional nine hospitals in Canada and nine more in

1 Neilos of Ancyra, quoted in Timothy S. Miller, "From Poorhouse to Hospital," *Christian History*, no. 101 (2011): 20, https://christianhistoryinstitute.org/magazine/article/from-poorhouse-to-hospital.

2 See Charles Gerard, *A Brief History of Hôtel-Dieu de Montréal: 1642–1942: The Second Oldest Hospital in Canada and the United States* (Catholic Hospital Association of the United States and Canada, 1942), https://www.chac.ca/documents/273/Montreal_Hotel-Dieu_de_Montreal_1642-1942.pdf.

the United States. Their intrepidness and faithfulness were the blueprint and inspiration for several other Catholic orders who also brought physical and spiritual healing to early settlements in the New World.

Fast forward to June 2023 in a land that was once home to a different Catholic missionary outpost in the New World. The Board of Regents of the University of California (UC) votes to end its affiliations with Catholic hospitals that abide by the Church's religious directives to affirm the dignity of human life at all stages of development. According to the vociferous protestations of activist groups, Catholic hospitals' prohibition of abortion, sterilization, artificial reproduction, physician-assisted suicide, and transgender treatments within their facilities marks them as intolerant and bigoted. The ire of California's sexual revolutionaries knows no limits when directed at the religious directives of Catholic hospitals—the state's largest providers of healthcare for the poor and underserved. In the defiant words of UC Board Chair John Pérez, "I don't think the number one research university (and) healthcare system in the country can say to women and LGBTQ+ people and those facing end-of-life issues, 'We just need you to jump a few extra hoops to get healthcare or we just need you to sacrifice a part of your humanity before you can be cared for here.'"[3]

The two vignettes presented above exemplify the harsh conditions that have faced Catholic healthcare over more than three hundred years in North America. While the continent's first missionaries had to contend with adverse natural conditions, the contemporary social and political climate toward the Church's mission of healing is unnaturally harsh and potentially more devastating to Christian ministries' ability to save souls. Indeed, the conceptions of the human person held by Christian anthropology and mainstream secular worldviews could not contrast more starkly.

What explains the pugnacious antagonism toward the Church's role in medicine by such cultural activists as the UC Board of Regents? Why would a public institution stifle the contributions of its state's largest provider of healthcare services for the poor and marginalized? The answer is revealed in the expression used by Pérez—suggesting that some people have to "sacrifice a part of [their] humanity" to receive care. The contemporary confusion about what confers humanity—or dignity—to all people lies at the root of modern American culture's rejection of Christian anthropology. Rather than recognizing the inherent dignity of human persons as an immutable aspect of being created by God, modern-day scolding secularists view the individual's self-definition as the ultimate

[3] John Pérez, quoted in Rania Soetirto, "UC Board of Regents Votes to End Affiliation with Restrictive Healthcare Institutions," *Daily Bruin*, June 27, 2021. https://dailybruin.com/2021/06/27/uc-board-of-regents-votes-to-end-affiliation-with-restrictive-healthcare-institutions.

source of the individual's dignity. For this reason, the Judeo-Christian definition of dignity is antithetical to the contemporary secular, self-referential understanding of the term.

When placed upon the arc of the Church's history and role in Western medical tradition, episodes such as the UC Board of Regents' actions seem wildly ahistorical. Indeed, the very ethos of Western medicine derives from the church teaching on the *imago Dei*: that the human person is created by God in his likeness and image. This revolutionary idea comes from the Judeo-Christian understanding of humanity's relationship to God. It stands in sharp contrast to the pagan beliefs of the pre-Christian Greek and Roman societies, which valued strength and wealth as being virtuous and did not see all people as deserving respect—or even life. The concept of *imago Dei* means that each human person reflects God the Creator, and thus the love that one shows to one's neighbor is akin to one's love of God. This profound realization motivated the early Christians in their tireless work on behalf of all suffering people in their midst, driven by the spirit of Christian charity and a desire to perform corporal works of mercy. Indeed, showing this intense love for God by caring for the suffering has animated Christian healing ministries ever since, the world over.

Understanding the Healing Arts in Pre-Christian Society

To grasp just how radical the concept of *imago Dei* was for early Christian communities, consider the pre-Christian understanding of philanthropy and the role of the healing arts within society. In ancient Greece, the concept of *philanthropia*—from which comes the word "philanthropy," meaning "a love of mankind"—described the relationship of the gods to humans. The presence of a power differential between *philanthropia*'s subject and object was implied in the term's usage: at its core, philanthropy describes a concern for humanity on a societal level. The term did not yet have a personal, individual meaning or refer to concern for the poor or weak, whose marginalized status was rather seen as confirming their inferiority.[4]

In ancient Rome, the word *humanitas* came to represent many of the same virtues of Greek *philanthropia*. As a quality marking the educated, *humanitas* was characterized by general sympathy and consideration for others, politeness, and social graciousness. For physicians, *humanitas* meant love of humanity was the prime motivation behind their care for the destitute as well as their advancement of

---

[4] See Gary B. Ferngren, *Medicine and Health Care in Early Christianity* (Johns Hopkins University Press, 2009), 86–87.

medical knowledge—surpassing love of honor, fame, and financial success. *Humanitas* was a principal condition of the role of the physician, as a member of the helping profession of medicine.[5]

The ancient world's concept of human dignity included the implicit notion that inequality among individuals and classes was part of society. Human rights were not inherent to the human condition, that is, but rather were associated with status or class. Individuals of highest standing—namely, those members of the upper class who demonstrated excellence in virtue—possessed the highest dignity and consequently were regarded as having the greatest worth.[6]

The classical world's precursors to the hospital—itself a Christian reflection of the concept of *imago Dei*—give insight into the meaning of human dignity in that world. In ancient Rome, *valetudinaria* were created to tend to ill and injured soldiers and slaves.[7] That these facilities' services were restricted to those with economic importance to the Empire—either as warriors or servants—underscored the material motives of these institutions.[8] The practice of invoking the intercession of the gods for healing in return for material offerings, performed in temples called *asclepieia*, grew out of ancient Greece and spread across the eastern Mediterranean, eventually reaching the Roman Empire. Spiritual healers promised cures for those who had the means to make a proper offering; the afflicted person was invited to sleep in the temple, where they would receive a divine vision that outlined a remedy for their ailments.[9] In contrast to later hospitals espousing the Judeo-Christian belief in universal human dignity as creatures created in the *imago Dei*, ancient Roman and Greek healing institutions were not based on a foundational assumption of the intrinsic value of every person, including those afflicted by disease or injury.

Early Christianity and Medicine

Underground communities of Christians who were dedicated to caring for the sick and poor out of selfless *agape* (love) for each person constituted a revolutionary development in the first few centuries AD.[10] From the early Christian communities of the first through third centuries, a

---

[5] Ferngren, *Medicine in Early Christianity*, 92–93.

[6] Ferngren, *Medicine in Early Christianity*, 95–96.

[7] Timothy S. Miller, *The Birth of the Hospital in the Byzantine Empire* (Johns Hopkins University Press, 1997), 38–39.

[8] Ferngren, *Medicine in Early Christianity*, 124.

[9] Ferngren, *Medicine in Early Christianity*, 136–37.

[10] Ferngren, *Medicine in Early Christianity*, 122.

disproportionate number of physicians emerged, drawn to imitate Christ the Divine Physician through their healing service.[11] Their love and care for the ill and destitute, even those who were not Christian, attracted large numbers of pagans to convert to the Christian faith. As a result, some historians estimate that the Church grew by as much as 40% per decade during its first three centuries.[12] One wonders whether this exponential growth through conversion came about because early Christian physicians were offering more effective healing, or whether it can be attributed to the love that the early Christian healers showed to those they served—those most disparaged as the outcasts of society.

With time, the clandestine early Church structured its healing mission into an organization that provided care for the poor, infirm, and abandoned in a manner inconceivable to the Roman ruling class. Throughout the Roman persecutions, as well as a pandemic (called the Plague of Cyprian) that decimated the Empire's population in the mid-third century, an organized group of Christian healers saw it as their spiritual obligation to care for the sick—and they risked infirmity and death to tend those afflicted by the plague. Responding to Christ's call to love their neighbor according to the parable of the Good Samaritan, these Christians extended their healing ministry beyond their coreligionists to include afflicted pagans as well.[13]

A towering pinnacle of Christians' organized exercise of works of charity—one that remains with us today—is the development of the hospital, an institution borne out of selfless Christian giving. Following Christ's teaching to love one's neighbor by serving the sick, early Christians administered charitable entities through their communities to assist greater numbers of people.

The earliest prototypes of the hospital appeared in the mid-fourth century, when St. Basil's monastic community near Caesarea, in modern-day Turkey, founded a *ptocheion,* a special institution dedicated to caring for the poor and sick as an expression of Christian charity. Unlike the ancient Greek and Roman healing centers of *asclepieia* and *valetudinaria,* which lacked several hallmarks of the hospital, Basil's almshouse offered room and board, round-the-clock nursing care, and the services of professional physicians to serve the sick. In addition to clinical care, Basil's *ptocheion* also offered accommodations for foreign travelers and societal outcasts, such as lepers.[14] In the saint's funeral eulogy,

---

[11] Mike Aquilina, *The Healing Imperative: The Early Church and the Invention of Medicine as We Know It* (Emmaus Road Publishing, 2017), 50–51.

[12] Aquilina, *Healing Imperative,* 59.

[13] Aquilina, *Healing Imperative,* 71–73.

[14] Miller, *Birth of the Hospital,* 50–53, 98–99.

St. Gregory of Nazianzus, Basil's close friend and successor to the bishopric of Caesarea, offered this praise for Basil's lasting legacy: "Go a little way outside the city to see a new city, the treasury of piety, a common treasure room of those who have possessions where superfluous wealth . . . is stored. . . . In this institution diseases are studied, misfortune made blessed, and sympathy put to the test."[15]

With time, the healing ministry established by Basil expanded to other cities and came to be regarded across Christendom as the mark of a caring and civilized society. In the centuries that followed, other metropolises, particularly across the East, modeled their hospitals after Basil's *ptocheion* and were seen as an indispensable asset that attested to the civic care of the poor and sick.[16]

Western Medicine in North America

To bring this reflection on the growth of Christian medical ministry closer to our own time and place, recall the harrowing achievements of the faithful, such as Mance and de Maisonneuve and their group of settlers in seventeenth-century Montreal who founded that outpost's hôtel-Dieu. The new-world expansion of Christian health services to serve the sick and poor was driven by a sense of social mission, which attracted faithful young people to join the religious life and to proclaim the Gospel to those they served. In the ensuing centuries, Catholic orders were prolific in establishing hospitals as extensions of their religious mission. For example, the Sisters of Charity, who first arrived in Baltimore, Maryland, to run that city's infirmary in 1827, went on to erect forty-four hospitals by the year 1898.[17]

In the late nineteenth and early twentieth centuries, Catholic hospitals in America went from being poorhouses, intended to shelter only the indigent, to respected centers of clinical and scientific inquiry. This transformation improved the public's perception of Catholic hospitals while contributing necessary financial and staffing resources to a burgeoning medical profession.[18] However, given that the US Catholic population

---

[15] Gregory of Nazianzus, quoted in Timothy S. Miller, "Basil's House of Healing: How a Fourth-Century Monk Pioneered the Hospital," *Christian History*, no. 101 (2011): 13.

[16] Miller, *Birth of the Hospital*, 85–87.

[17] Peter J. Levin, "Bold Vision: Catholic Sisters and the Creation of American Hospitals," *Journal of Community Health* 36, no. 3 (June 2011): 343–47.

[18] Gail Farr Casterline, "St. Joseph's and St. Mary's: The Origins of Catholic Hospitals in Philadelphia," *Pennsylvania Magazine of History and Biography* 108, no. 3 (July 1984): 289–314.

at the time grew mostly through immigration, most Catholic communities were substantially poorer than their non-Catholic, US-born counterparts. The funding challenges for Catholic hospitals then meant that a small number of paying patients subsidized the charity care provided to larger numbers of hospitalized patients.[19]

Events of the mid-twentieth century saw the effects of secularization reach Catholic hospitals in the United States. The complexity of healthcare economics ushered in by the new government programs such as Medicare and Medicaid in the mid-1960s heightened the challenges that Catholic hospitals faced in carrying out their charitable ministries. In the decades that followed, a more restrictive regulatory environment forced hospitals to drive down costs by reducing lengths of stay and adopting new business strategies to remain competitive. The result of these changes in healthcare finance and regulation was that Catholic hospitals began to rely more on lay administrators with business savvy, not boards of directors comprising men and women religious, to navigate the turbulent waters of American healthcare. This change in leadership composition—that is, from religious to secular—also had a deleterious effect on the perceived spiritual mission of Catholic hospitals in America, blurring the distinction between secular and religious healthcare systems in the public imagination.[20]

The expansion of third-party payors and the growing governmental regulation of healthcare coincided with a decline in religious vocations among the nuns and brothers who formed the backbone of Catholic healthcare ministries. Following the Second Vatican Council in the mid-1960s, various forces combined to result in fewer men and women religious; these forces included an exodus of religious from their orders, a trend toward smaller Catholic families, and a reduction in new vocations to religious life. Between 1960 and 1990, the numbers of religious sisters in the United States dropped nearly 40%, from 168,527 to 103,269, while the numbers of brothers plummeted from 10,473 in 1960 to a mere 6,743 thirty years later.[21]

The secularizing trend affecting American medicine since the mid-twentieth century mirrors, in large part, the overall secularizing trend seen in the broader society over the past eight decades. As the number of Americans professing religious affiliations has waned, so has the common understanding of the Judeo-Christian precepts upon which the country was founded. One casualty of the large-scale abandonment

---

[19] Casterline, "St. Joseph's and St. Mary's," 292.

[20] Barbra Mann Wall, *American Catholic Hospitals: A Century of Changing Markets and Missions* (Rutgers Press, 2016), 4–6.

[21] Wall, *American Catholic Hospitals*, 4.

of religious adherence in the US has been the respect for the religious mission that lies at the heart of Catholic medical ministries. With secular forces overtaking the health professions, louder, more strident voices have questioned the legitimacy of Catholic healthcare ministries' freedom to adhere to Catholic bioethical principles. Speaking of the healthcare directives of the United States Conference of Catholic Bishops (USCCB), Patricia Grabow notes, "The myriad prohibitions in care lead to the question, 'What enables a group of less than 300 Catholic bishops to define the healthcare of millions of Americans, 80% of whom are not Catholic?'"[22]

The pointedness of such questions illustrates the widespread lack of understanding of the First Amendment to the US Constitution, which gives pride of place to protecting the free exercise of religion. As more Americans divest themselves from a religiously informed worldview, the country's religious sensibilities continue to weaken. The loss of religious consciousness makes challenges to the legitimacy of religiously motivated organizations seem like reasonable arguments in an ostensibly pluralistic society.

Unfortunately, even many US Catholics are swayed by the arguments confronting their coreligionists in healthcare. With the secular worldview's overwhelming success in usurping any need for a spiritual anchor to maintain legitimacy, Americans of all (and no) religious backgrounds could be forgiven for treating religious viewpoints as an afterthought—a relic of a bygone era. The absence of faith principles in societal awareness can be attributed, among Catholics, to poor catechesis, leading to low awareness of church teaching on morals and social tradition. This unfamiliarity with Christian principles accelerates the emergence of a society that conducts itself without acknowledging God.

This chapter has examined how Christianity's bold claims about inherent human dignity—and the abundant charity of Christian healers through the centuries—formed and informed the Western medical tradition. I have also considered why the Christian imagination has lost prominence in our secularized (and secularizing) society. To reintroduce Christian social principles into healthcare—and to imagine a Catholic response that can reclaim the purpose of medicine—chapter 2 starts by unpacking the principles of Catholic social teaching and how they apply to the healing arts.

---

[22] Patricia A. Grabow, "Catholic Healthcare Delivery in America—Noble Origins to the Modern Era," American Association for Physician Leadership, December 17, 2023, https://www.physicianleaders.org/articles/catholic-healthcare-delivery-in-america-noble-origins-modern-era. See also USCCB, *Ethical and Religious Directives for Catholic Health Care Services*, 6th ed. (USCCB, 2018), http://www.usccb.org/about/doctrine/ethical-and-religious-directives/upload/ethical-religious-directives-catholic-health-service-sixth-edition-2016-06.pdf.

CHAPTER 2

Catholic Social Teaching and Its Application to the Healing Arts

"Each individual person has been created to love and to be loved."

—St. Teresa of Calcutta[1]

The Church has offered her moral instruction to the faithful on matters of social concern since the time of our Lord's earthly ministry. Simply put, this application of the Church's teaching to social issues—commonly called Catholic social teaching—addresses "the rights and duties of men organized into society."[2] Drawn from both Scripture and Tradition, the teachings of the Church govern Catholics in our personal, civic, and social lives, because no aspect of life lies outside the domain of the Lord of the universe.

Catholic social teaching is theological. Although its principles are often selectively cited to bolster particular ideological positions, sincere reflection on their instruction with an open heart reveals reasoning that defies the logic of humankind's political labels of liberal or conservative, left or right. While the theological principles at the heart of the Church's teachings on social and economic matters can be traced back to the earliest foundations of the Church, modernity posed new challenges in the nineteenth century that led to the poignant articulation of Catholic social teaching by Leo XIII in his landmark papal encyclical, *Rerum novarum*.

In *Rerum novarum*, Leo XIII responded to the crescendo of corporate capitalism that was buoyed by the dehumanizing aspects of the Industrial Revolution, as well as the countervailing forces of socialism that sought to rebuke the excesses of industrialization through conflictual class struggle. In this encyclical, he calls out the abuses to human dignity found in these competing economic models, while he also asserts the

---

1 St. Teresa of Calcutta, quoted in Susan Conroy, *Praying with Mother Teresa: Prayers, Insights, and Wisdom of Saint Teresa of Calcutta* (Marian Press, 2016), 34.

2 Thomas Storck, *An Economics of Justice and Charity: Catholic Social Teaching* (Angelico Press, 2017), 1.

rights of individuals to a broad distribution of private property acquired through the fruits of their labor, as well as to the family's right to control its means of subsistence. He speaks against robber barons' exploitation of the working masses, who were subject to poor labor conditions, injury, and illness in return for meager subsistence wages. He also denounces the excesses of any state that attempts to subvert the primacy of the individual and the family. In a challenge to adherents of both economic models, Leo XIII enjoined capitalists to recognize their duties to ensure workers are paid a living wage, and he commands socialists to see that socioeconomic classes can "dwell in harmony and agreement, so as to maintain the balance of the body politic."[3]

Catholic Social Teaching and Its Application to Medicine

While Leo XIII wrote *Rerum novarum* to address the political and social situation of his time, a careful reader of this prescient encyclical finds timeless lessons that apply the dilemmas of the present day, including those involving the delivery of medical care. Many people consider Catholic social teaching to be limited to matters of economics, social structure, and social function. As matters of social concern, medicine and the delivery of healthcare are fittingly assessed through the lens of Catholic principles. After all, the profession of medicine is a common good and an ethical enterprise; in this sense, the social teaching of the Church serves as an antidote to our contemporary culture's wholesale conversion of healthcare into a commodity that is subsidized by some governments. Given the social and economic dimensions of medicine, the application of Catholic social teaching to medical care necessarily works to establish the common good and a more just culture. Put another way, the manner in which society cares for its sick reflects the measure to which it applies justice and the common good.

Human Dignity

In secular discourse today, popular appeals to the concept of human dignity are common. Like many other words that are debated in the popular lexicon, the exact usage of the term "human dignity" in relation to Catholic teaching differs from what most people understand in vernacular usage. When infused with our culture's outsized reliance on individual

---

[3] Leo XIII, *Rerum novarum*, no. 19.

autonomy, secular references to dignity often imply a self-referential definition, rather than a universal principle.

In many common contexts, the word "dignity" is used to connote a right to self-actualization. In these times, when a self-referential definition of values is deemed the highest good, human dignity is sometimes erroneously promoted by creating self-proclaimed rights to actions that the Christian recognizes as belonging solely to God. Examples include autonomy over choosing when one will die, decisions to continue to nurture a pregnancy (or not), and the expectation that others ought to refer to us by how we define ourselves. By this criterion, the preservation of human dignity may even imply that others are obliged to affirm concepts that violate observable reality (think "preferred pronouns") or to act in opposition to one's own idea of dignity (such as the expectation that physicians participate in the legalization of physician-assisted suicide in the name of "death with dignity," as is the case in some jurisdictions across the Western world). These self-referential definitions also imply that human dignity is not absolute but rather conditional, with some people having more "dignity" than others, in keeping with a secular humanist, utilitarian view of human worth (e.g., based on conditions such as "consciousness" or "quality of life").

The Christian Meaning of Human Dignity and Its Importance in Medicine

As discussed in the preceding chapter, one of the most radical propositions of the Judeo-Christian worldview is the idea that all human beings are made in the image and likeness of God—*imago Dei*. Thus, the very essence of our nature as humans entails an irrevocable self-worth that cannot be erased. It is ours because we are creatures created by God, and all people are called to be God's children. Moreover, this concept of human dignity characterizes all people at all stages of life, irrespective of any other condition.

Perhaps nowhere else in society is this *imago Dei* concept of human dignity more significant than in medicine. As a pillar of medical ethics, the idea that all human beings possess inviolable worth defines the profession's obligation to promote and protect all human life and to support human flourishing at all stages of development. This is why we say that a doctor who cares for a pregnant woman has two patients: the woman and her unborn child. It is why the AMA is right to condemn physicians' participation in executions. It is why it is wrong for anyone, particularly physicians, to promote the killing of the unborn—in the womb, in the case of abortion, or in a petri dish, in the case of in vitro fertilization. The inviolable worth of humans means that doctors may not "play God" in choosing whether to carry out their professional duty to preserve and restore human life. The absolute nature of human dignity, as understood by Christians, is perhaps best summarized by Pope Francis: "Promoting the dignity of the person means recognizing that he or she possesses inalienable rights which no one may take away arbitrarily."[4]

Solidarity

One of the cornerstones of Catholic social teaching is the principle of solidarity. What does this mean in practical terms? And how does this apply to healthcare? Does the principle of solidarity have any relevance to how Christians seek out (and how Christian medical personnel provide) medical care?

The concept of solidarity in Christian teaching is based on the idea that all are called to care for one another, as sisters and brothers living in society. Justice and charity demand that we work together to secure the protection and well-being of other members of our community, with special attention to those who are vulnerable or marginalized. As St. John Paul II defined it, solidarity is "a firm and persevering determination to commit oneself to the common good; that is to say to the good of all and of each individual, because we are all really responsible for all."[5]

"Now that all sounds very good," you might say, "but how does this concept apply to medical care in a society like the United States, where public assistance and social welfare programs exist to care for the poor?"

Since the mid-twentieth century, the United States has developed a sizable social safety net to account for the healthcare needs of materially poor Americans. Over recent decades, this safety net has expanded to include an ever-larger segment of the US populace. At their inception in 1965, the Medicare and Medicaid programs were promoted to provide assistance to the elderly and to poor Americans in need of medical services. Over the years, the number (and percentage) of the US populace enrolled in these programs has expanded; they are no longer last-ditch rescue programs reserved for a small segment of marginalized Americans. To cite one example, as of 2023, Medicare and Medicaid made up 21% and 18% of all US healthcare expenditures, respectively—the second- and third-highest-spending entities after private health

---

4 Francis, Address to the European Parliament, November 25, 2014, https://www.vatican.va/content/francesco/en/speeches/2014/november/documents/papa-francesco_20141125_strasburgo-parlamento-europeo.html.

5 John Paul II, Encyclical *Sollicitudo rei socialis* (*For the Twentieth Anniversary of "Populorum Progressio"*), December 30, 1987, no. 38, https://www.vatican.va/content/john-paul-ii/en/encyclicals/documents/hf_jp-ii_enc_30121987_sollicitudo-rei-socialis.html.

insurance.[6] The 2010 ACA, as well as the relaxing of Medicaid eligibility requirements and the government's freeze on Medicaid disenrollments during the COVID-19 emergency, served as inflection points in greatly expanding the numbers of Americans covered by these programs. In short, rather than being backstops for a small segment of Americans who have fallen on hard times, public welfare programs have come to be viewed as an entitlement upon which larger swaths of the US population depend to meet basic needs.

Returning to the concept of solidarity, remember that Christian solidarity, in its most authentic form, is a matter of personal responsibility. Our responsibility to exercise Christian solidarity is not satisfied by declaring it the duty of government to meet the needs of the poor. Elected officials and bureaucrats may craft public assistance programs, but these do not substitute for the demonstration of true solidarity with those in need by men and women with faces, hands, and hearts. A pernicious effect of the overgrowth of public programs is that along with the growth of welfare programs comes a diffused sense of responsibility on behalf of ordinary citizens to care for their neighbors. In fact, the creation of regulations to oversee such bureaucratic organizations often creates obstacles to providing true Christian charity. An example is the accusations of fraud and federal law violations levied against physicians for waiving copays or deductibles for patients enrolled in Medicare.

When exploring the effects of public assistance on solidarity, the case can also be made that, far from benefiting ordinary citizens, the government and insurers undermine the average working family's ability to afford basic medical care. Following this line of thinking, the encroachment of public payors (and commercial insurance payors) over the whole US healthcare system is one leading contributor to the unaffordability of basic services for ordinary Americans. This effect occurs when these government programs dictate payment schemes (e.g., how much service providers will be paid for a given service) as well as establish the regulatory mechanisms that determine payment conditions. Because such processes—that is, payment controls and regulatory oversight—are decoupled from the costs of providing services, and from patients' true need for the services, the cost of healthcare tends to be inflated when the government plays a larger role in healthcare financing and price fixing.

Sadly, one factor that has contributed to driving US primary care into the ground has been the very government programs that ostensibly provide access to a larger segment of the US population. The increase in practice overhead needed to comply with the rules and regulations—not

---

6 US Centers for Medicare and Medicaid Services (CMS), "NHE [National Health Expenditure] Fact Sheet," modified December 18, 2024, https://www.cms.gov/data-research/statistics-trends-and-reports/national-health-expenditure-data/nhe-fact-sheet.

to mention the payment amounts dictated by programs (sometimes, in the case of many Medicaid plans, less than the cost of providing care)—has forced many independent primary care practices to sell out to larger health systems in order to survive. This consolidation has worked in turn to the detriment of working-class Americans who lack private insurance and do not qualify for public assistance. In essence, advocates of expanding Medicaid, Medicare, and government-subsidized insurance take a position that forces more people to depend on state assistance for even the most basic medical services, such as primary care.

Government public assistance therefore differs from the Christian notion of solidarity in three fundamental ways:

1. Government programs are incapable of acting as authentic expressions of solidarity because they are, by definition, run by faceless and nameless bureaucratic institutions. They lack the capacity to build human relationships and exhibit compassion, which is the cornerstone of solidarity.
2. Public assistance programs are themselves a sort of political currency. Their expansion and funding are used as levers of control to promote desired social outcomes—a far cry from solidarity's foundation on justice and charity.
3. Rather than serve as a temporary assistance for needy individuals who are struggling to access medical care, far-reaching government programs promote intergenerational dependence on government. Expanding the numbers of people who depend on public assistance means that fewer people can provide for their own needs without relying on government programs—which itself undermines the dignity one derives from work and from meeting one's own needs and the needs of the family.

In contrast, a Christian approach to primary medical care provides care for the vulnerable and marginalized in the local community. One way we can respond to this need is by offering working-class people care that is economically accessible, while also offering care to materially poor people who would not otherwise be able to access medical services. By viewing solidarity as a starting point, Christian primary care practices prioritize economic accessibility and welcome for the vulnerable as expressions of justice and charity. I describe detailed examples of practices exhibiting such qualities in chapter 7.

Subsidiarity

A second core tenet of Catholic social teaching is the principle of subsidiarity. Like the two principles already discussed—dignity of the human person and solidarity—the principle of subsidiarity is intricately connected to the other Catholic social teaching principles. That is, one cannot discuss subsidiarity without a clear understanding of its relationship to both solidarity and the dignity of the human person.

For starters, consider what subsidiarity means. The *Catechism of the Catholic Church* defines subsidiarity in the following way: "The teaching of the Church has elaborated the principle of *subsidiarity*, according to which 'a community of a higher order should not interfere in the internal life of a community of a lower order, depriving the latter of its functions, but rather should support it in case of need and help to co-ordinate its activity with the activities of the rest of society, always with a view to the common good.'"[7] In other words, subsidiarity states responsibilities and decision making properly encourage participation in, and take place at, the lowest appropriate tier of community life—without interference from higher tiers beyond that which is necessary to fulfill a function. Contrary to some assertions, subsidiarity is not an antigovernment principle. For example, some functions are best carried out by higher levels of the government (e.g., national defense, interstate law enforcement) that would be ineffective or disastrous if left to lower levels of government or the community. In sum, the proper application of subsidiarity—like the principles of solidarity and dignity of the human person—is directed toward the advancement of the common good.

With specific regard to medical care, the concept of local control has been largely abandoned in favor of health system consolidation, uniformly applied algorithmic practice protocols, medical documentation, and payment infrastructure that has homogenized the way care is delivered. What's more, the infiltration of the public health concept of "population health" into the lexicon of medical education for student doctors has further eroded the most subsidiarity-based relationship in medicine: the doctor-patient relationship. The rationale for these forms of standardization and collectivism in medicine is based largely on the idea that healthcare is too expensive and complex to be managed successfully at a local level—in other words, that some economy of scale is needed to realize the cost containment and efficiency necessary to deliver care across a country as large as the United States.

This assumption includes a category error, namely, that cost and complexity mandate a higher order of management over the administration of medical care. This error supposes that "healthcare" is a monolithic entity that is best managed and financed with similar mechanisms

---

7 *Catechism of the Catholic Church*, 2nd ed. (United States Conference of Catholic Bishops, 2016), no. 1883, citing John Paul II, Encyclical *Centesimus annus* (*On the Hundredth Anniversary of "Rerum Novarum"*), no. 48 §4; see also Pius XI, Encyclical *Quadragesimo anno* (*On Reconstruction of the Social Order*) I, 184–186.

across all aspects of medicine. The reality is that different disciplines of medicine are inherently distinct in regard to the resources and personnel each discipline needs to function, as well as to the volume and circumstances of the demand for each. As an example, primary care is, by definition, most people's entry point into the medical system. The need for primary care is often predictable and routine, and the services it provides are relatively inexpensive compared to other specialty care. On the other hand, services such as trauma care and intensive care are used by far fewer people, are more unpredictable, and cost more to provide. Therefore, the financing models for such specialized disciplines ought to differ from the financing model for primary care.

By making these three care domains—the primary care office, trauma bay, and intensive care unit—reliant on the same insurance-based model, the system drastically inflates the cost of primary care and severely limits the ways care can be provided. Rather than burden primary care practices with the hefty overhead and confining regulation inherent in insurance participation, decoupling primary care from insurance and governmental payors would actually free physicians and patients from encumbrances and limitations imposed by those third parties. Following the principle of subsidiarity, such decoupling could restore primary care decision making to the level of the doctor and patient—the lowest (and most appropriate) level of management in this most intimate of human interactions. Decoupling primary care from third-party payments would work hand in hand with solidarity by conferring to local agents the responsibility for the medical needs of people in the community, and it would respect the dignity of the person by making primary care more accessible to all people, irrespective of whether they carry an insurance card. (In cases where a social safety net is necessary, patients—rather than state bureaucracies—ought to be the main decision makers about the way resources are allocated.)

Locally rooted practices that respond to local conditions and the needs of patients. An economic model that decentralizes care and allows patients and doctors to take ownership of care. A practice model that does not exclude anyone on the basis of insurance networks or employment status. In summary, this is what subsidiarity in primary care medicine looks like.

Stewardship of Resources

The Catholic social teaching principle of stewardship reminds us that human beings have a duty to safeguard God's creation. Although this principle is often applied to our relationship to the natural environment, the same principles can apply to all resources bestowed by God for human flourishing. Just like natural resources such as air, water, and land, other gifts like human talents, material, and financial resources are

God-given and ought to be employed in a way that respects their provenance from the Most High, as well as their natural end to further the common good—not only supporting those living today, but also keeping in mind the welfare of future generations.

Extrapolating this thinking to how resources are used in the development and delivery of medical care, note that several types of resources are required to provide such care. Financial investment, material resources, and human ingenuity and intelligence go into the development of diagnostic tests, treatments, and techniques that promote human health and healing. We should all be profoundly grateful for the bountiful gifts that produce such innovations for the purpose of restoring and preserving health.

However, to anyone who has interacted with the healthcare system, it is obvious that the delivery of healthcare is permeated with a vast amount of wastefulness. The medical field is consumed by an overgrowth of regulation, resulting in byzantine payment models and delivery mechanisms that inevitably lead to great waste of money and the diversion of human talents. This waste occurs in service to bureaucratic and managerial functions that perpetuate many systems and practices that do nothing to advance the ostensible aim of the healthcare system: treating and curing illness and furthering health.

Add the vast workforce of functionaries who are removed from actual patient contact by orders of magnitude, and the result is an inflation in the cost of care and a diffusion of responsibility for the function (or dysfunction) of the system. This increased cost is baked into the price of goods and services produced by the healthcare apparatus. Governmental payors (namely, Medicare and Medicaid) place caps on what they will pay for services; commercial insurers negotiate rates with service providers (doctors, hospitals, and the like). Only the uninsured patient is made to bear the list price of the medical care provided to him. In other words, the very people who are least able to pay the full "sticker price" of medical care are the ones who must negotiate on their own behalf with the healthcare provider (hospital, clinic) to resolve the inflated charges for which they are held responsible.

In light of Catholic social teaching, the scenario described above is a tremendous affront to the principle of stewardship on many levels. First, this system is not a prudent or judicial use of the economic or material resources given by God to promote health. A recent study found that up to 30% of US healthcare spending was spent on administration, and at least half of administrative spending was wasteful.[8] Aside from wasteful

---

[8] "The Role of Administrative Waste in Excess US Health Spending," *Health Affairs*, October 6, 2022, https://www.healthaffairs.org/content/briefs/role-administrative-waste-excess-us-health-spending#:~:text=Research%20indicates%20that%20the%20US,OECD%20nations%20plus%20the%20US.

spending, a large contingent of people hold positions that serve primarily to maintain the existing system's bureaucratic infrastructure without directly benefiting patient care. One could argue this bureaucracy represents a misapplication of human resources that could better serve the care of patients in some other way, or be directed toward some other pursuit outside healthcare—think of retraining large numbers of billing auditors and referral coordinators to assume clinical roles in patient care.

Another way that the current healthcare system works against the principle of stewardship has to do with how the system applies financial resources. To capture revenue from governmental payors and commercial insurance plans, provider organizations must ensure adherence to measurable metrics and protocols. Administrative functions that are designed to comply with these directives result in higher prices for medical care—and they skew the aim of care from solely focusing on the patient to focusing on regulatory and financial mandates. This system works against the common good by diverting resources away from real care, inflating the cost of care, and increasing the dependence of individuals and families on third-party payors to supply and pay for all their healthcare needs. In Catholic social teaching parlance, the current system also undermines subsidiarity (i.e., local control in decision making) and solidarity (i.e., the joining of justice and charity), in detriment to the common good.

How can we reverse some of the poor stewardship inherent to the prevailing healthcare system? For one, bear in mind that modern medicine is not monolithic—it comprises a multitude of disciplines offering care in a variety of clinical settings. The material and personnel needs of distinct specialties and care settings are markedly different—think of the needs of a primary care office versus those of a liver transplant service.

Unfortunately, the prevailing insurance-dependent economic model that currently finances nearly all healthcare expenses has plundered economic and organizational resources in primary care. The reason is manifold. First, primary care is not an "insurable" event in the same way trauma or emergency room care is—unlike emergency room care, most primary care is predictable and foreseeable. Most people expect to see their primary care physician a handful of times per year for preventive care, a random episode of acute illness, or monitoring of chronic conditions such as diabetes and hypertension. In contrast, people generally do not anticipate having a major medical event, such as a heart attack or stroke, that leads to an ER visit or hospitalization.

The second way in which the insurance-payment model has hurt primary care is by treating the primary care practice as a loss leader. This assumption means that large healthcare systems prefer to treat their primary care practices as financial liabilities, existing for the purpose of driving patients toward more lucrative services and specialties. The enormous overhead costs imposed on primary care practices—responsible for such tasks as requesting insurance authorization for subspecialty referrals, imaging studies, and the like—make these practices appear to operate at a loss. For primary care practices owned by larger healthcare systems, referrals for ancillary services such as labs and imaging are routed internally within the larger system as a means to control the cost of the service.

The refocusing on stewardship in primary care is best achieved by decoupling primary care from large multispecialty health systems, whose financial interests are at odds with primary care's goals to minimize and prevent hospital-based and specialty care. I would go a step farther to argue that true primary care stewardship would entirely sever the financial relationship to the insurance- and government-payment mechanism. Because of its relatively predictable and low-cost nature, primary care ought to be accessible to the average American without resorting to the prepaid money laundering scheme by which the insurance industry operates in tandem with monopolistic healthcare systems. The goals of primary care are opposite to those of the hospital system—at its best, primary care obviates the need for higher-level medical care, whereas hospital-based care tends to incentivize more costly care. Even newer schemes such as "value-based care"—the newest iteration of the failed managed-care policies of the 1990s—face a large burden of regulatory costs and metric-driven protocols that work at cross-purposes.

The Catholic social teaching principle of stewardship is therefore intimately related to the principles of human dignity, solidarity, and subsidiarity. When applied in a primary care context, stewardship promotes human flourishing through a judicious use of economic and human resources in promoting the common good—relying on local autonomous control over the care delivery, in response to the demands of justice and charity.

Summary

This chapter has taken the thirty-thousand-foot view of Catholic social teaching and considered how four of its foundational principles apply to the medical profession: namely, the Catholic understanding of the dignity of the human person, solidarity, subsidiarity, and stewardship. And I have dispelled some common yet erroneous positions held by those who bend the Church's social doctrine to accommodate preconceived political or social agendas.

For the next chapter, keep these principles in mind as we prepare to hold them up as a yardstick to assess some prevalent practices and beliefs of the present-day US healthcare system.

CHAPTER 3

The Contemporary American Healthcare System Viewed Through the Lens of Catholic Social Teaching

"I intend now and at all times to venerate in everyone the image of God, in whose likeness they were created."

—St. Vincent Pallotti[1]

Chapter 2 examined the fundamentals of Catholic social teaching and how they can apply to the profession of medicine. In this chapter, I consider the current state of medicine and healthcare delivery from the perspective of these same Catholic principles. While many aspects of such a critique may seem facile—particularly regarding the frequently cited life issues of human sexuality and procreation—the prevailing medical culture regularly opposes authentic expression of Christian principles in myriad other ways.

My motive for such an analysis is not to engage in cultural hand-wringing, political disparagement, or doomsday prognosticating about the future, but rather to face, with clear eyes, the challenges that confront us. We are an "Easter people," as St. John Paul II exhorted us, and we must always resist the temptation to despair.[2] Yes, the cultural tide of the present moment has shifted decisively against those of us who wish to live our faith in ways that shine its light into every aspect of our lives. Nevertheless, we must never become despondent, never yield to anxiety about whether we will succeed in declaring victory over the culture. As the great St. Teresa of Calcutta so famously said, "God has not called me to be successful. He has called me to be faithful."[3]

---

1 Vincent Pallotti, quoted in Vensus George, *Find the God Who Seeks You: Journeying with St. Vincent Pallotti, the Prophet of Communion* (Catholic Apostolate Center, 2011).

2 John Paul II, Angelus, Apostolic Journey to the Far East and Oceania, November 30, 1986, https://www.vatican.va/content/john-paul-ii/en/angelus/1986/documents/hf_jp-ii_ang_19861130.html.

3 Teresa of Calcutta, quoted in Phyllis Theroux, "Amazing Grace: Mother Teresa Comes to Anacostia," *The Washington Post*, October 18, 1981, https://www

With that disclaimer, let us proceed with this analysis.

The traditional understanding of medicine as a profession has been mischaracterized and distorted in recent decades, in parallel with the coarsening and secularization of society at large. As the great ethicist and physician Edmund Pellegrino noted, these societal trends "are exacerbated by the de-professionalization of medicine, which views health care as a commodity, and its delivery as a matter of corporate enterprise, profit, and commercialization."[4] As the larger culture has deposed the truth of faith and has instead given pride of place to a pervasive hyperindividualism, discourse about ethics and morality in the public square—particularly surrounding issues of life and human procreation—is now considered an outdated and tired exercise from an antiquated era and an obstacle to individual self-realization. Thus, in contemporary public discourse, the right to life has been supplanted by the right to "reproductive freedom"; the defense of sanctity at the end of life has been met with the "death with dignity" movement; and efforts to prevent the destruction of human life created in the laboratory are trampled by the steady march of self-determination declared through the growing recourse to in vitro fertilization and other assisted reproductive technologies (ART).

To the faithful Christian, all these examples are glaring violations of our call to respect and protect the God-given dignity of every human person. That our society has shown such contempt for strident attempts by the faithful to defend life is further proof that the culture has become untethered from the Judeo-Christian worldview upon which it was founded. This lack of adherence to a common moral norm has resulted in a lack of understanding of the accompaniment of faith and reason in addressing moral questions. This lack of understanding in turn opens space for confusion that distorts the truth as it applies to a right-ordered moral order. These distortions regarding life issues in medicine pose attacks on authentic human dignity, even as they masquerade as substitutes.

The triumph of the individual has led to the secular belief that the highest good is determined by the autonomous self. Our society's abandonment of God in the common discourse has resulted in a de facto atheistic public square. We no longer acknowledge any obligation toward God on an individual or societal level. Rather, the morality of an individual's actions is determined solely by what the individual can do and chooses to do and by whether the individual has the consent of others visibly affected by those actions.

.washingtonpost.com/archive/lifestyle/magazine/1981/10/18/amazing-grace/80c3d328-1270-4f50-90d8-ba72dc903b90/.

[4] Edmund D. Pellegrino, *The Philosophy of Medicine Reborn: A Pellegrino Reader* (University of Notre Dame Press, 2008), 283.

Attacks on the Dignity of the Person

Christians understand that human dignity derives from being created in God's image and likeness—summed up as *imago Dei*. Examples of the contemporary medical culture's assault on the *imago Dei* abound. These are seen most obviously in issues related to the genesis of the human person, procreation, and sexuality. Despite great strides in scientific understanding of human physiology and disease, authoritative voices in the medical community have sidestepped scientific reason regarding human development, choosing instead to adopt social theories that place individual autonomy at the pinnacle of the ethical pyramid.

This denial of scientific truths was not always the order of the day. In fact, the scientific perspective on the beginning of human life has long acknowledged its origin in fertilization. As one modern scientific textbook of embryology explains, "Human development is a continuous process that begins when an oocyte (ovum) from a female is fertilized by a sperm (spermatozoon) from a male to form a single-celled zygote."[5] This science-informed reasoning explains why many physicians commonly hear in their training that the doctor who cares for a pregnant woman is charged with preserving the health of two patients: the mother and her unborn child.

Sadly, mainstream thought leaders in the medical community no longer engage with the question of a physician's duty to preserve and promote preborn human life. In their position statements on abortion and artificial reproductive technology, secular professional journals and medical specialty societies that claim to speak for American physicians foreclose even the possibility of dialogue with their physician colleagues and constituents who assert the preeminent Hippocratic duty to safeguard all human life from the earliest stages of development. Instead, prominent thought leaders in these organizations reframe such issues in terms of unrestricted individual autonomy. They exploit the sacrosanct nature of the doctor-patient relationship, using it as a shield to obfuscate discussions about the moral standing of unborn human life. As a case in point, Jack Resneck Jr., then AMA president, commented on the US Supreme Court's 2022 *Dobbs v. Jackson Women's Health Organization* decision, which overturned legalized abortion at the federal level. He said the ruling represents "an egregious allowance of government intrusion into the medical examination room, a direct attack on the practice of

---

[5] E. V. N. Persaud and Mark G. Torchia, *The Developing Human: Clinically Oriented Embryology*, 12th ed. (Elsevier, 2025), 1.

medicine and the patient-physician relationship, and a brazen violation of patients' rights to evidence-based reproductive health services."[6]

The medical establishment's treatment of in vitro fertilization and other ART follows a similar logic, elevating to supreme importance the individual's right to self-determination at the expense of any responsibility toward the unborn children who are manufactured in laboratories. In February 2024, the Alabama Supreme Court's decision in *LePage vs. The Center for Reproductive Medicine and Mobile Infirmary Association* applied the law equally to born and unborn children regarding wrongful death claims. In response, Verda J. Hicks, then president of the American College of Obstetricians and Gynecologists (ACOG), declared that "the outcome of this case will certainly affect access to fertility treatment across the country as more and more state legislatures advance policies that are based on an ideological and unscientific definition of personhood."[7] By issuing this attack on the concept of personhood, the ACOG president seems to have conceded that the embryo is human and does possess life. However, by charging that claims of an embryo's personhood are "unscientific" and "ideological," she—like other mouthpieces for mainstream medical associations—sidesteps any discussion of when the developing human deserves protections by ACOG constituent physicians. In this way, medical authorities morph their arguments to accommodate their changing definitions of key terms such as "personhood" and "human life."

A similar vocabulary manipulation is taking place in the redefinition of human sexuality that promotes newly evolving ideologies that advance the concept of gender as distinct from biological sex, the belief that gender exists on a spectrum, and the proposition that sex is changeable. In contrast to the Christian belief that men and women are imbued with dignity by God and that their sexuality is immutably determined by their Creator, social activists who advance LGBTQ+ ideology rest their argument on the notion that the "dignity" of the individual rests solely on his or her self-definition. Not only does the individual today define the concept of dignity, but by virtue of considering such dignity dependent on self-definition and therefore "fluid," one may revise and redefine the concept at any future point. Furthermore, this false notion of dignity is claimed to be offended when the larger society or other individuals refuse to accept such a self-definition.

---

[6] Jack Resneck Jr., quoted in "Advocacy in Action: Protecting Reproductive Health," American Medical Association, May 31, 2024, https://www.ama-assn.org/delivering-care/public-health/advocacy-action-protecting-reproductive-health.

[7] Verda J. Hicks, quoted in "ACOG Statement on Alabama Supreme Court IVF Decision," news release, American College of Obstetricians and Gynecologists, February 21, 2024, https://www.acog.org/news/news-releases/2024/02/acog-statement-on-alabama-supreme-court-ivf-decision.

From a Catholic Christian perspective, such a view has many serious problems. First, the concept that humans have a gender distinct from biologically determined sex promotes a form of dualism that is contrary to the Christian understanding of the human person. As Archbishop Alexander Sample of Portland, Oregon, clearly stated in his 2023 resource titled *A Catholic Response to Gender Identity Theory*, the dualist ideas advanced by gender ideology deny God's will in the created order, reject the goodness of his gift in the form of our bodies, and instead root "sexed identity in a dissociated self-perception rather than the body."[8] The idea that people are free to change their sexual identity to align with their perceived gender represents an outright rejection of God's creation of each person in his image as a man or woman.

One of the greatest scandals in modern US medicine has been the full-throated promotion of gender ideology by mainstream medical associations. Against all generational wisdom and the observable reality of humans' existence as male and female, the purported scientific experts have rushed to adopt a formulation of gender theory that is neither scientific nor historical. Medical specialty societies have partnered with activist organizations to write clinical guidelines based purely on this ideological framework. These pronouncements include glossaries of terms such as "trans woman," "cis gender," and "assigned at birth" to provide cover for linguistic deceptions. As Mary Hasson so clearly states, "Gender ideology has gained a foothold in culture by obscuring the truth that the human person exists as an embodied male or female person from the moment of conception."[9] The introduction of new terminology and distorted conceptualizations of human sexuality, promoted by mainstream medical societies, harms people afflicted by treatment decisions that are legitimized by this false ideology, and it challenges Catholic medical professionals who attend to people who suffer from its distortions.

Consider one example of this false view of human sexuality and social activism, couched and promoted in the language of the sacrosanct doctor-patient relationship by medical specialty societies. Specifically, the American Academy of Family Physicians (AAFP) has asserted that "diversity in gender identity and expression is a normal part of the human existence and does not represent pathology. The AAFP supports

---

8 Alexander K. Sample, *A Catholic Response to Gender Identity Theory: Catechesis and Pastoral Guidelines for the Archdiocese of Portland in Oregon,* January 25, 2023, https://files.ecatholic.com/12494/documents/2023/1/EN_A%20Catholic%20Response%20to%20Gender%20Identity%20Theory_FINAL2023.pdf.

9 Mary Hasson, "Corrupting Language, Creating Confusion," in *Gender Ideology and Pastoral Practice: A Handbook for Catholic Clergy, Counselors, and Ministerial Leaders,* ed. Theresa Farnan, Susan Selner-Wright, and Robert L. Fastiggi (En Route Books and Media, LLC, 2024), 431.

access to gender-affirming care for gender-diverse patients, including children and adolescents." The AAFP policy statement goes on to advocate that "the full spectrum of gender-affirming care should be legal and should remain a treatment decision between a physician and their patient."[10] Sadly, the AAFP is no outlier when it comes to antiscientific declarations in support of gender ideology and clinical interventions that disfigure the healthy, properly functioning bodies of patients suffering with gender dysphoria. The American Academy of Pediatrics, the American College of Physicians, and the American Association of Clinical Endocrinology all have adopted policy statements that cloak the fallacy of gender ideology in the guise of scientific legitimacy.[11] The ideological capture of US medical institutions threatens the profession's ability to promote authentic human dignity in accord with Christian anthropology and Hippocratic principles.

Although life issues in medicine offer the most evident examples of secular medicine's attack on authentic human dignity, the delivery system and its economic structure also undermine the dignity of both patients and physicians. Over the past several decades, with the growing influence of both governmental and commercial third-party payors, physicians have been strong-armed into surrendering their clinical and prudential judgment regarding how they care for patients. The strengthening of the financial muscle of third parties has coincided with clinical associations' rising expectations of adherence to clinical algorithms as "standard of care." These trends have resulted in the subtle assertion that physicians are interchangeable, inasmuch as physicians are expected to apply clinical guideline algorithms uniformly and nearly without exception. The implementation of these clinical protocols is subject to the approval of formularies developed by third-party payors, whose control of the purse strings subjects every doctor's medical recommendation to payor approval. Whether a physician's prescription is

---

[10] "Care for the Transgender and Gender Nonbinary Patient," American Academy of Family Physicians, September 2024 COD, https://www.aafp.org/about/policies/all/transgender-nonbinary.html.

[11] See "AAP Reaffirms Gender-Affirming Care Policy, Authorizes Systematic Review of Evidence to Guide Update," American Academy of Pediatrics, August 4, 2023, https://publications.aap.org/aapnews/news/25340/AAP-reaffirms-gender-affirming-care-policy; "ACP Updates Guidance to Promote Health Equity for LGBTQ+ Patients," American College of Physicians, July 12, 2024, https://www.acponline.org/advocacy/acp-advocate/archive/july-12-2024/acp-updates-guidance-to-promote-health-equity-for-lgbtq-patients; "AACE Position Statement: Transgender and Gender Diverse Patients and the Endocrine Community," American Association of Clinical Endocrinology, March 7, 2022, https://pro.aace.com/recent-news-and-updates/aace-position-statement-transgender-and-gender-diverse-patients.

authorized is largely determined by negotiated business deals among insurance and pharmaceutical companies—two forces that wield unbridled control over Americans' financial access to care.

Rote protocols pose other concerning problems for medical decision making. The application of narrow, "evidence-based" clinical algorithms to broad swaths of patients—because they happen to share a common clinical condition, despite other important differences in their health profiles—neglects individual distinctions. The expectation that these clinical algorithms will be applied wholesale to categories of patients overrides individual clinical judgment by physicians who must assess the appropriateness of care in light of the metric-driven protocols that dominate US healthcare. The damaging effects of this protocol-based uniformity of care become magnified as increasing numbers of physicians practice as employees of larger healthcare entities, which demand obeisance to company policies and the expectations of payors.

Whether through eliminating distinctions between physicians and other clinical staff or through failing to consider individual patient differences when applying care metrics, the erasure of variants among practitioners and patients represents an affront to the human dignity of both clinicians and the people they care for. It replaces the ideal of a profession with a consumerist transactional model, wherein the patient is merely a customer and the physician a mere purveyor of services. The outcome of such a model is the degradation of human dignity—both of patients who are suffering and of the medical professionals they consult for help.

The Erosion of Solidarity

As mentioned in chapter 2, the Christian concept of solidarity addresses a calling to care for all and offer support for all. Solidarity is the charge given to each individual Christian to assume responsibility for his or her neighbor in a local, personal way. As St. John Paul II explained in his encyclical *Sollicitudo rei socialis*, solidarity "is not a feeling of vague compassion or shallow distress at the misfortunes of so many people, both near and far. On the contrary, it is a firm and persevering determination to commit oneself to the common good; that is to say to the good of all and of each individual, because we are all really responsible for all."[12]

The personal nature of Christian solidarity, rooted in love of neighbor, belies the common misunderstanding that expanded government social programs can stand in for personal responsibility. Advocates for enlarging public welfare projects characterize the government as a benevolent caretaker with responsibility for the basic material needs

---

[12] John Paul II, *Sollicitudo rei socialis*, no. 38.

of the citizenry. Those who see the growth of public programs as an extension of solidarity overlook the fact that the government is nothing more than a faceless bureaucratic institution, incapable of caring for, or expressing concern for, anyone. Care and compassion are capacities that can be expressed only by individuals toward other persons; public organizations can determine how resources are to be allocated, but these entities do not have the capacity to care, to empathize, or to love. Our Lord did not call us to adopt a vague, sentimental love of humankind. Rather, as we read in John 13:34–35, Jesus states, "I give you a new commandment, that you love one another. Just as I have loved you, you also should love one another."

Within contemporary medicine, another misconception related to the principle of solidarity derives from its conflation with population health in clinical care and medical education. The term "population health," coined in 1990 by Robert Evans and Greg Stoddart,[13] is defined as "the health outcomes of a group of individuals, including the distribution of such outcomes within the group."[14] The focus on population health emphasizes social, environmental, and economic factors, collectively described as determinants of health. Although medicine has long recognized the impact of environmental factors on individuals' health, the sleight of hand found in the population health movement undermines the integrity of the medical profession.

Allow me to explain.

The expanding concept of population health has redirected the focus of the medical profession away from what was once its singular concern: the fiduciary duty of the physician to the individual patient sitting in front of him or her. The change in treatment focus from individual to population paralleled changes in the way healthcare was financed in the mid-twentieth century, as insurance and public payors assumed an increasing role in paying for medical care. The existential threat that this shift poses to the traditional ethos of medicine cannot be overstated, because to foment confusion regarding the doctor's primary loyalty is to sabotage the very nature of the profession itself. This shift confuses the aims of the medical doctor who is caring for an individual patient with the objectives of the public health official tasked with promoting the health of the community, and with the goals of the insurance actuary

---

[13] R. G. Evans and G. L. Stoddart, "Producing Health, Consuming Health Care," *Social Science Medicine* 31, no. 12 (1990): 1347–63, https://doi.org/10.1016/0277-9536(90)90074-3.

[14] Mina Silberberg, Viviana Martinez-Bianchi, and Michelle J. Lyn, "What Is Population Health?" *Primary Care* 46, no. 4 (December 2019): 475–84, https://doi.org/10.1016/j.pop.2019.07.001.

whose job it is to assess financial risks on behalf of a payor.[15] In deciding which policies to promote, the public health professional must calculate the collective balance of risks and benefits; the actuary thinks of the financial risk to the company. The physician, on the other hand, owes full allegiance to the well-being of the person who has come for help. The doctor's exam room is reserved for the single-minded advancement of the authentic flourishing of the patient. Often, individual social factors play an outsize role in the management of the patient's condition; but the duty to advocate on behalf of the individual patient must never be confused with the sentimental activism of social progress.

Another contentious feature of the push for population health has to do with the vocabulary used to promote it. One can scarcely read any treatment of population health without wading into a discussion of the social determinants of health—that is to say, those social, economic, and political factors that "determine" the health outcomes of individuals and populations. This use of the word "determinant" connotes a fatalistic definitude, as though one were trapped in an inevitable life circumstance from which escape is impossible. It suggests that these social factors—such as poverty, educational attainment, or even residential postal codes—will destine those affected to poor health outcomes. Common sense and experience support the premise that social adversity opposes good health and human flourishing, but it does not follow that individuals are powerless or stripped of agency in overcoming these obstacles. Furthermore, the perceived inevitability of poor health outcomes among individuals who face social factors categorized as adverse social determinants is wielded to justify medical associations' adoption of social policies that encourage clinicians to view patients first and foremost through the lens of demographics. In a nutshell, the rationale behind these policies argues that the unequal social circumstances of certain categories of people demands that the medical profession bear responsibility to deliver equal outcomes for demographic groups that are deemed disadvantaged. In reality, much of these outcome disparities are related to factors outside the purview of medical care. And while the medical profession is duty bound to a social contract to promote the common good, this obligation does not replace the physician's primary responsibility—that is, to act in the best interest of the individual patient—with efforts at social engineering.[16] For the Catholic medical professional, this

---

[15] See Michel Accad, *Moving Mountains: A Socratic Challenge to the Theory and Practice of Population Medicine* (Green Publishing House, 2017), 103.

[16] See Richard L. Cruess and Sylvia R. Cruess, "Professionalism, Communities of Practice, and Medicine's Social Contract," in "Special 50th Anniversary Issue," supplement, *Journal of the American Board of Family Medicine* 33 (September 2020): S50-S56, https://doi.org/10.3122/jabfm.2020.S1.190417.

duty is manifest in the commitment to see the face of Christ in each person who presents for care.

For these reasons, the expanding concept of population health as an inseparable aspect of the clinical care of patients presents challenges to the Christian understanding of solidarity. The next chapter discusses the linguistic ploys represented by terms like "population health" and "evidence-based medicine."

The Undermining of Subsidiarity

In the past century, Americans have become accustomed to an enlarged role of government in their everyday lives. Perhaps nowhere has this increasing scope been more evident than in the way we conceptualize and receive medical services, with the creation of public programs and insurance subsidies as means to organize and finance the ever-enlarging health services sector. Healthcare programs such as Medicare and Medicaid, and insurance subsidies through the ACA, together accounted for nearly a quarter of the US federal budget in 2023 at $1.6 trillion—nearly double the federal spending on national defense.[17]

It was not always this way. In the first part of the twentieth century, most Americans paid relatively modest fees for medical services from their personal checkbooks. Ensuing years saw the genesis of employment-based, employer-financed provision of medical care in the United States. In 1938, the businessman Henry Kaiser collaborated with a physician group to provide prepaid medical services to thousands of construction workers on the Grand Coulee Dam for the cost of seven cents per worker per day. Wage controls implemented during World War II led to the proliferation of employer-sponsored health insurance as part of benefits packages to attract new workers, becoming a perennial staple of employment arrangements.

Then in 1965, President Lyndon B. Johnson signed legislation that established Medicare and Medicaid as means to provide medical care for those who are elderly, poor, and disabled.[18] Growth of these programs over time—along with the 2010 enactment of the ACA and its government-subsidized insurance marketplaces, as well as the expansion of several state Medicaid programs—has entrenched the federal and state

---

[17] Juliette Cubanski et al., "FAQs on Health Spending, the Federal Budget, and Budget Enforcement Tools," KFF, March 20, 2023, https://www.kff.org/medicare/issue-brief/faqs-on-health-spending-the-federal-budget-and-budget-enforcement-tools/.

[18] See Michael J. Zinner and Kevin R. Laughlin, "The Evolution of Health Care in America," *The Urologic Clinics of North America* 36, no. 1 (February 2009): 1–10, https://doi.org/10.1016/j.ucl.2008.08.005.

governments as de facto guarantors of Americans' access to healthcare. By legislative fiat, lawmakers have imposed a top-down mechanism that governs the financing and regulation of medical services and provides upward pressure that distorts the cost of medical products and services. In addition to usurping control of medical care from local service providers, these programs' bureaucratic demands impose additional administrative costs that disproportionately burden small practices. These administrative and financial pressures are partially responsible for the rapid decline in the number of independent medical practices. In 2022, the share of physicians practicing in physician-owned practices dropped to 46.7%, down from just over 60% a decade earlier.[19]

Expanding government control over the practice of medicine has cumulatively all but eradicated the notion of subsidiarity within the profession. Whereas in times past physicians believed that their oath and the social contract required them to provide a certain amount of pro bono care for the economically disadvantaged, the pervasively expanding nature of government assistance programs such as Medicaid has changed physicians' calculus around providing care to those who are indigent. The incremental growth of public programs among a larger swath of patients, combined with the programs' relatively low reimbursement levels, has altered the social contract and added economic tensions for physicians in independent practice, which in turn has weakened physicians' relationships with their patients.[20] In essence, by shifting responsibility to care for the poor from individuals to faceless public programs, the government has diluted the sense of shared accountability, making care access a matter of public policy rather than a personal moral duty.

The effect of these changes on US primary care has been pernicious and unrelenting. Decoupling patients from the immediate financial impact of their care—combined with the strained ties of social responsibility, as downstream effects of the government's expansion across healthcare—has led the cash price of even modest primary care services to rise beyond the reach of the average working family. The administrative overhead required for a practice to maintain compliance with the leviathan regulatory requirements of third parties has also fueled the increased cost of primary care. This price inflation and the minimal essential coverage requirements required by the ACA have reinforced the assertion that third-party payors are essential to provide most

[19] Ericka L. Adler, "Trends in Buying and Selling Medical Practices," *Medical Economics*, March 4, 2024, https://www.medicaleconomics.com/view/trends-in-buying-and-selling-medical-practices.

[20] See Darcy Nikol Bryan, "A Physician's Perspective," in *The Economics of Medicaid*, ed. Jason J. Fichtner (Mercatus Center at George Mason University, 2014), 99–125.

Americans with access to health services. The negative feedback loop of a zero-sum approach to healthcare access impoverishes the public imagination about how to make medical care more effective and accessible, undermining local initiatives to create grassroots solutions that meet the most basic medical needs of people in their local communities. Failure to differentiate between primary care (such as the local family doctor's office) and highly specialized, procedural care (such as the intensive care unit, surgery, and trauma service) in the financial model that now funds healthcare services has neutered the former's effectiveness and rendered it a loss leader within the byzantine medical-industrial complex of American healthcare.

The complementary natures of solidarity and subsidiarity in pursuing justice within the healthcare system is evident given that an affront to one of these principles necessarily prevents the natural function of the other. Solidarity is harmed by depersonalizing our individual responsibility to care for our neighbor in a personal and local way. Transferring that obligation to faceless bureaucracies and public programs further distorts individual Christians' understanding of their duties—as citizens and as Christians—through subsidiarity. In a similar manner, overgrown and monopolistic top-down command of healthcare delivery and financing disrupts local efforts to solve the problems of medical access, thereby also harming the principle of subsidiarity. The near total control of healthcare by federal legislation and agencies has other pernicious effects on the ecology of healthcare. The wastefulness of this approach lies at the root of contemporary American medicine's assault on another key Catholic social principle: the effective stewardship of resources.

The Assault on Good Stewardship of Resources

Historically, the Church has spoken mainly about the Christian duty to exercise effective stewardship in relation to ecology and the natural world. As the modern world has become more complex, and the political and economic aspects of society have become more intertwined, the Church's call for responsible stewardship has expanded to encompass other social goods and resources that support the Christian understanding of human dignity and a harmonious and just society. Conceptualizing medical care as a fundamental need in a just society makes it a key resource in need of effective stewardship in a right-ordered community.

The growth in US healthcare spending is on track to outpace the gross domestic product (GDP) into the next decade, increasing the percentage of GDP spent on healthcare to 19.7% in 2032. In 2023, healthcare spending rose 7.5%, outpacing the GDP rise of 6.1%; this increase made national health expenditures amount to 17.6% of the nation's

GDP.[21] For Medicare alone, the average per capita expenditure exceeded $15,700 in 2023, resulting in a total government Medicare outlay of $848.2 billion—or 14% of the nation's $6.2 trillion annual budget.[22] For the 153 million people on employer-sponsored health insurance in 2023, the average annual premium was $8,435 for single coverage and $23,968 for family coverage, representing a 7% year-over-year increase.[23]

The centralization of financial control of the healthcare system has made federal health spending ripe for wastefulness and abuse. By some estimates, upwards of 30% of US healthcare spending is directed to administrative costs.[24] Meanwhile, the US Government Accounting Office has estimated that improper payments (meaning errors and fraud) from the Centers for Medicare and Medicaid Services (CMS) exceeded $100 billion in 2023.[25] When it comes to health outcomes, the return on this investment is embarrassingly poor. In recent years US life expectancy has worsened compared to peer countries; in 2022, for example, US life expectancy was 77.5 years, compared 82.2 years in peer countries. Other measures, such as premature death, are also higher in the United States, with higher rates of child and adolescent deaths from motor vehicle accidents, firearms, and suicide among the principal causes.[26]

Clearly, the economic cost and trajectory of spending on healthcare in the United States—not to mention the tragic preventable loss of life and increased morbidity—are neither desirable nor sustainable. They represent a tremendous waste of the nation's economic treasure—garnered from American workers' hard-earned wages and tax payments—as well as an impoverishment of health and life as a result of a wasteful

---

[21] Jacqueline A. Fiore et al., "National Health Expenditure Projections, 2023–32: Payer Trends Diverge as Pandemic-Related Policies Fade," *Health Affairs* 43, no. 7 (June 12, 2024): 910–21, https://doi.org/10.1377/hlthaff.2024.00469.

[22] "How Much Does the Government Spend on Healthcare?" USAFacts, updated August 1, 2024, https://usafacts.org/articles/how-much-does-the-government-spend-on-medicare/.

[23] Kaiser Family Foundation, *Employer Health Benefits 2023 Annual Survey* (KFF, 2023), https://files.kff.org/attachment/Employer-Health-Benefits-Survey-2023-Annual-Survey.pdf.

[24] *Health Affairs*, "Excess US Health Spending."

[25] US Government Accountability Office, "Medicare and Medicaid: Additional Actions Needed to Enhance Program Integrity and Save Billions" (GAO-24-107487, April 16, 2024), https://www.gao.gov/products/gao-24–107487.

[26] Emma Wager et al., "How Does the Quality of the U.S. Health System Compare to Other Countries?" Peterson-KFF Health System Tracker, October 23, 2023, https://www.healthsystemtracker.org/chart-collection/quality-u-s-healthcare-system-compare-countries/.

and dysfunctional system. Such wastefulness demonstrates poor stewardship and constitutes an assault on justice and the common good.

The national debate over how to improve healthcare outcomes and control spending has been a long-standing staple of US political cycles. On one side of the debate are those who advocate for a larger role for government in managing and administering healthcare. They claim that the only just way for the country to reduce costs and obtain outcomes on par with peer countries, such as those in most of Western Europe, is to expand government spending and control. On the other side are those who challenge the notion that expanded government will result in a more efficient and higher-functioning healthcare system; they point to cost controls and rationing, as well as the usurping of individual choice in the government-run healthcare bureaucracies of many peer countries. They also point to government wastefulness in administering resources as a prime reason why greater governmental control over healthcare is undesirable.

From the standpoint of a Christian response on how best to structure a societal approach to healthcare access, the issue is largely a prudential one for which Catholic social teaching offers practical insight. Faithful Christians of goodwill have come down on both sides of the debate about the government's role in preserving access to medical care. For this book's purposes, I focus more specifically on how a just society might best direct resources to ensure access to the services that primary care provides.

It is folly to adopt the same financial model for the provision of primary care that applies to financing more specialized care that requires a higher level of resources, such as intensive care or trauma surgery. An analogy can be drawn to the financing of home repairs. While we expect that people resort to their homeowner's insurance policy to finance rebuilding after a natural disaster, they would seem foolish if they demanded that insurance cover basic anticipated maintenance, such as changing air filters or repairing a cracked window. In the same way, disconnecting primary care from the overburdened, overregulated, and costly mechanism of insurance micromanagement would reduce the cost of primary care services for all. The exclusion of primary care from the essential health benefits of comprehensive insurance plans would also reduce insurance premiums for the average enrollee. Moreover, removing the constraints that third-party payors impose on primary care physicians' clinical decision making would increase physicians' freedom to practice as they see fit—and empower patients to choose physicians based on factors other than their participation in insurance networks. In other words, an increase in local control (rather than governmental control) and personal stewardship (rather than federal budgetary control) for primary care is a prudential Christian response to the burgeoning bureaucratic and fiscal intrusion on US primary care.

The prevailing medical system's disregard for the dignity of the human person, its evisceration of the principles of solidarity and subsidiarity, and its wastefulness in plundering vast resources on a national and individual level—taken together, these make it hard to know where to begin an attempt to change things. The problems are so intractable that a more feasible strategy would be to construct an alternate, parallel system that honors Hippocratic medicine and a Christian anthropology. Part of shedding the old system involves recognizing how embedded we have become in its way of thinking. And nothing reflects the mindset of the current medical paradigm as much as language. I examine how language shapes our thinking in the next chapter.

CHAPTER 4

The Importance of Language in the Takeover of Medicine

"Far be it from us to be seduced with the fair promises in which Satan is sure to hide his poison! Do you think he is so unskilful in his craft, as to ask you openly and plainly to join him in his warfare against the Truth? No; he offers you baits to tempt you. He promises you civil liberty; he promises you equality; he promises you trade and wealth; he promises you a remission of taxes; he promises you reform. . . . He shows you how to become as gods. Then he laughs and jokes with you, and gets intimate with you; he takes your hand, and gets his fingers between yours, and grasps them, and then you are his."

—St. John Henry Newman[1]

Thus far, this book has looked at the importance of healing ministry in spreading Christianity and at how Christians have shaped the ethos of the medical profession. I also reviewed principles of Catholic social teaching and how these principles apply to the practice of medicine. Then the preceding chapter examined contemporary medical culture through the lens of Catholic social teaching, including examples of the mainstream healthcare establishment's violations of human dignity, its undermining of true Christian solidarity and subsidiarity, and how it obliterates any notion of effective stewardship and the common good rooted in justice.

How did the profession of medicine diverge so greatly from its original purpose and the spiritual underpinnings that shaped it? What forces allowed those opposed to medicine's deep Christian roots to undermine its guiding compass? To be sure, the co-opting of the medical profession is part of a larger ideological takeover affecting the whole of the West. Hence, this question is much broader than can be answered in this book.

[1] John Henry Newman, Lecture 1, "The Times of Antichrist," in *Discussions and Arguments on Various Subjects*, 3rd ed. (Pickering and Co., 1878), 60–61.

However, one strategy by which the disruptors of medicine's tradition sow confusion involves the deceptive use of language to obfuscate and distract. Not unlike other areas of public life, leaders in medicine are more concerned with being discredited by the zeitgeist and less fearful of abandoning the truth, even scientific truth. To avoid criticism in the court of public opinion, mainstream medicine's leadership success relies on accepting the terms of the public discussion by redefining words and creating neologisms to frame the debate. In this brief chapter, I shed light on basic assumptions and techniques that medicine's thought leaders employ in their quest for ideological control of medicine—techniques far from the time-honored values of the the Christian origins of Western medicine and the Hippocratic tradition that preceded it.

One of the broadest assumptions that secular medical associations make—promulgating the assumption as a matter of professional consensus—is the insistence that physicians remain neutral on ethical matters in their professional roles. In deference to the notion of all-encompassing patient autonomy, so the thinking goes, the medical professional's highest duty is to further the patient's wholly autonomous demands. This chapter explores and dissects this idea, which I refer to as the "myth of the neutral physician."

I also take a magnifying glass to the language employed by mainstream medical mouthpieces in their attempt to define terms that place any discussion of contemporary healthcare in terms favorable to their ends. As in other spheres, control of the language defines the terms of debate, largely predicting who will be viewed as holding the higher ground. Usually, these linguistic sleights of hand are so skillfully performed as to be nearly imperceptible to critics, and thus are they adopted and propagated by opponents. For this reason, we must recognize how everyday language has become part of the battleground of ideas surrounding the culture of medicine. Calling out this tactic and refusing to use imprecise language that misrepresents medicine's *telos*, rightly understood, are imperative if we are to learn how to resist ideological takeover and raise the awareness of both our colleagues and the public about medicine's true purpose and function.

The Myth of the Neutral Physician

The prevailing secular medical ethos idealizes the morally neutral physician. In contemporary medical thought, physicians and other medical professionals are free to hold personal positions on any number of clinical ethical matters, so long as they do not allow those personal beliefs to interfere with their patients' rights of autonomy. This widely held belief is the primary argument against a broad recognition of physicians' rights of conscience, perhaps nowhere better articulated than in Ronit Y. Stahl and Ezekiel J. Emanuel's 2017 article "Physicians, Not Conscripts" in the *New England Journal of Medicine*. The authors asserted that physicians have a duty to participate in interventions that, in their view, are not "medically controversial" as defined by the AMA. They press even further by declaring, "Health care professionals who are unwilling to accept these limits have two choices: select an area of medicine, such as radiology, that will not put them in situations that conflict with their personal morality or, if there is no such area, leave the profession."[2] This worldview—in which the AMA is the final arbiter of medical ethics—affords no place for physicians who dissent from its secular orthodoxies, and thus it offers no care options for patients who wish to enlist the services of a physician who aligns with their deeply held ethics if those ethics diverge from the AMA's settled conclusions.

According to the mouthpieces of mainstream medical organizations, there can exist no debate about issues upon which they have declared a consensus. Their consensus opinion is thus deemed to be the neutral default position; those who do not acquiesce must be ideologues who allow personal morality to interject itself in the exam room, violating the highest secular good of absolute patient autonomy. These same thought leaders fail to recognize the forced morality imposed by a medical establishment that has erased generations of cultural and societal consensus on professional ethical norms. The regular violation of physician rights of conscience has profound consequences for doctors and patients alike, and it is one of the most compelling arguments in favor of the development of what I am calling Benedict Medicine.

Language as Deception in Medicine

In the molecular biology laboratory, a plasmid is an independent, self-replicating strand of DNA that encodes information the scientist wishes to be expressed in the cell. This segment of genetic material can be used to alter a cell's DNA composition. The researcher introduces the DNA sequence into the host cell, where it is incorporated and replicated as part of the cell's genetic makeup. Thus, editing the structural "language" of the cell becomes a sort of biological Trojan horse, surreptitiously presenting a string of data that becomes incorporated permanently into the cell's makeup.

So too, the introduction of novel definitions and neologisms fundamentally alters the way society communicates. Recent decades have

---

2 Ronit Y. Stahl and Ezekiel J. Emanuel, "Physicians, Not Conscripts—Conscientious Objection in Health Care," *New England Journal of Medicine* 376, no. 14 (2017): 1380–85, https://doi.org/10.1007/s11017-025-09703-8.

brought a slew of new terms and expressions that rewire perceptions of commonly held ideas and disrupt shared understanding. The field of medicine is rife with examples of these linguistic plasmids, some of which I explore here.

Ranking highest among words most despised among physicians in clinical practice is the word "provider." This word has become ubiquitous in the American lexicon, used in the medical and lay press and even in medical education as shorthand to raze distinctions between physicians and clinicians with other levels of training, such as physician assistants and nurse practitioners. The wholesale practice in which corporate medicine labels all clinicians "providers" has largely succeeded in leveling the differences between individuals and their professional titles, in communications with both their medical staffs and the public. Magnifying the word "provider" leads to the deprofessionalization of the role of the physician in clinical care. Such a generic word de-emphasizes the differences, in experience and training, that exist between physicians and other clinical professionals.

In addition to diminishing these differences, the term "provider" substantiates the commercial aspect of modern healthcare. After all, if the system runs on the work of providers, what are these providers providing? Are they providing health, or healthcare? Are they merely service providers whose only role is technical, like those who work at the cable company or who bus a table at a restaurant? And if there are providers, then surely there must be "consumers" who use the services being provided. (Medicine historically has referred to these consumers as "patients.") The noxious effect of such terminology is clear when one considers that bright young medical students rarely aspire to become providers—however, many dream of someday becoming doctors. (That said, when reviewing medical students' applications for residency training, occasionally I do come across a student's essay that describes a desire to become a "provider"—a self-inflicted wound and immediate red flag that the student has succumbed to this nefarious denegation of his or her chosen profession.)

A variation on this theme—more specifically targeting primary care—is the abbreviation PCP as shorthand for "primary care provider." In some circles, this abbreviation is said to refer to primary care physicians. However, when the term is used in settings where "provider" predominates, it is a distinction without a difference. In any event, PCP as the abbreviation for the recreational drug phencyclidine seems to have been forgotten by nearly everyone in healthcare administration.

In fairness, healthcare leadership has made some attempt, albeit half-hearted, to assert a distinction between physicians and other clinicians. This forced attempt has given us the acronym APP, for advanced practice provider. In healthcare administration, APP refers to any clinician who is not a physician (usually physician assistants and nurse practitioners). While this neologism may convey meaning in health system board meetings, it is poorly understood by the general public. The people in the clinic waiting room may be forgiven if they assume that the advanced practice provider they are seeing today holds some special qualification that their physician does not. My point in bringing up these new monikers is not to inflame the debate about the merits or demerits of these newer clinical roles, but rather to make the case that these new labels ultimately deprofessionalize physicians in the clinical landscape.

Another term unique to the healthcare industry (not to be confused with the medical profession) is the word "reimbursement." While other sectors of the economy refer to "payments" or "fees," medical financing has created a system where the norm is to delay payment by third parties for services rendered. By calling physician payments "reimbursements," medical economists have distanced physicians' economic activity from that of other sectors of the economy. The term "reimbursement" obscures the pricing of medical services because the amount paid depends not on a set price for everyone, but instead on backroom contracting between service providers and payors. This opacity is why health systems' charge masters quote "rack rates" that are exorbitantly high—when the insurance company negotiates a lower rate, patients' explanations of benefits make them believe their insurance company is saving them money. Since the ACA's mechanisms incentivized the consolidation of medical practices, smaller independent medical practices have operated at a distinct disadvantage when it comes to negotiating reimbursement rates and maintaining the overhead needed for them to comply with the proliferation of regulations and documentation required to prove their quality of care. Which leads to the next topic.

The "Quality" and "Value-Based" Boondoggle

Two words that often appear together in the medical literature serve as masterful linguistic Trojan horses: "quality" and "value." To reframe the rules of engagement within the industry, healthcare gurus have gone on the offensive by asserting their own meanings for these two powerful words. They have co-opted the virtue-laden idea of quality by equating it with adherence to their predefined set of metrics; these often include levels of performing certain preventive interventions or prescribing specific medications that are indicated for particular medical conditions. Sometimes the definition of "quality" hinges on the number of patients with favorable outcomes on those interventions or screening tests. That is, if a practitioner's patient panel scores poorly overall on a specific disease-monitoring parameter, this outcome is seen as evidence of dubious quality. These measurements of so-called quality serve as a sort of social credit system, allowing third-party payors and public-facing watchdog organizations to sort "providers" by their performance on these quality metrics.

Closely tied to quality is the concept of value. In the rubric of healthcare leadership, the definition of "value" encompasses care quality (as defined above) as well as provider performance and patient experience.[3] The inclusion of these last two components attempts to incorporate the perceptions of patients and the practice patterns of clinicians. However, the limited variables used to define "value" in healthcare calls to mind Henry Ford's quip about the Model-T: "Any customer can have a car painted any color that he wants so long as it's black."[4] The same can be said about healthcare quality and value.

Physicians as Mini-Public Health Experts

In my considerable time as a physician in academic practice, I have seen a noticeable shift toward the concept of population health, which creates tension with medicine's primary focus on the individual patient. As mentioned in preceding chapters, this change in priorities is premised on the idea that physicians play a critical role in containing healthcare costs and achieving the broader vision of healthcare equity—a term that lacks a firm definition but nonetheless yielded more than thirty-four thousand articles on the topic in a simple search I conducted in PubMed, the medical literature database, in March 2025.

On the surface, entrusting physicians with increasing the public's consciousness about rising costs related to prescribing and practice patterns seems like a positive trend. If that were all that the system were proposing, this innocuous stance would even seem to support the principle of effective stewardship of resources, as discussed in chapter 2. The difficulty arises when physicians are saddled with the tension between this responsibility for population outcomes and their traditional role as uncompromised advocates for the well-being of the individual patient in the exam room. When physicians' clinical judgment is pitted against cost containment or some other value, the result is a catch-22 from which clinicians cannot escape unscathed. Either they sidestep the demands for cost containment and act purely in the fiduciary role as patient advocates—putting them at odds with the function of the system—or they

---

3 CMS, "Value-Based Care," updated February 27, 2025, https://www.cms.gov/priorities/innovation/key-concepts/value-based-care.

4 Henry Ford with Samuel Crowther, My Life and Work (Doubleday, Page & Company, 1922), https://archive.org/details/mylifeandwork00crowgoog/page/n10/mode/2up.

compromise their duty to patients in favor of the outside pressures of cost containment and panel metrics.

Since the inception of Western medicine, physicians have made the care of the individual patient their ideal. Recall from chapter 1 that the Hippocratic oath, dating to at least the third century BC, establishes as much. And while the medical profession has looked favorably at understanding the patient's environment as an important aspect of understanding the patient's condition, in recent decades the profession has begun take on an increasingly activist role in shaping that environment after its own image. Today's push for an increased focus on populations has less to do with improving the conditions of individual patients and more to do with a coordinated project of social engineering, in which the medical profession is just one player. The stridency of medical associations in promoting population health as a means to so-called health equity—itself closely tied to the political regime that focuses more on aggregate outcomes of demographic groups than on the needs of the individual patient—reveals the utopian vision to which medical leaders are adherents. (Population health and its use as a tool for political activism were discussed in greater detail in chapter 3.)

Finally, the concept of evidence-based medicine (EBM) is conceptually related to population health, in that it relies on aggregate data to drive treatment recommendations. The evidence-based paradigm analyzes the outcomes of studies of large cohorts of subjects (in meta-analyses, randomized controlled trials, and systematic reviews) to determine how interventions affect outcomes of a statistically significant number of test subjects. As the numbers of people studied grows, the likelihood of individual benefit from the intervention becomes smaller. Thus, EBM is useful for predicting the effects of interventions on an average sampling of the population being studied, but it is not as useful for predicting the effects of interventions on individual patients. Because of this discrepancy between aggregate effects and individual outcomes, EBM is an unwieldy tool for the individual clinician to use in the treatment of her or his individual patient. Overreliance on EBM in developing clinical care guidelines and algorithms disproportionately applies the results of population studies to individuals, giving such population-level outcomes outsize importance in directing the personal physician's care of the patient in the exam room.[5]

[5] See Accad, *Moving Mountains,* 106–11.

Summary

These examples mentioned in this chapter are but a small sampling of ways in which medicine has been ideologically captured on a broad scale. As Christian medical professionals, we should be aware of the linguistic traps that have been set for us, as well as the conceptual pitfalls inherent in the unchallenged maxims of population health and evidence-based medicine. Adopting the mental models and preferred lexicon of the insurgents undercuts the primacy of the doctor-patient relationship and Christian anthropology as supported by science. Relinquishing this territory is a form of surrender; it abandons true solidarity with the distressed patient who comes to us for care and authentic compassion.

Part II

A Manual for Reclaiming the Telos *of Medicine*

CHAPTER 5

Building the Frame of Benedict Medicine

"Jesus Christ presents each of us with a challenge and a call. Will we step out of the boat to walk on the waves with him? Will we leave everything to follow Christ? The problem with too many Catholics is that we have forgotten this primary call to discipleship and have settled for a religion in which there is no risk, no call and no challenge."

—Fr. Dwight Longenecker[1]

Part one of this book contemplated the rich history of Western medicine as a manifestation of its *telos*, or purpose. This reflection on the primary principles of Catholic social teaching and their application to the practice of medicine lays bare the ways in which contemporary American healthcare has warped the exercise of the profession, turning against Western medicine's Christian origins. This analysis critiques modern medicine's incoherence by explicating how the secular industrial concept of healthcare diverges from medicine's deeply spiritual and transcendental origin and meaning.

While we could content ourselves with purely theoretical analyses of this theme (the type that is usually confined to academic writing), our calling as Christians is more practical. We are compelled to strive to integrate all aspects of our lives—to manifest in the world the truth we have come to know through faith and reason. In other words, we are urged to put into practice what we have seen and learned and to share it with others. Hence, part two of this book offers a practical manual to consider how we might restore the true intention of medical practice and wield it as an instrument for bringing the truth to those around us. The vision of medical care as a spiritual endeavor in turn leads to the strengthening of more vibrant Christian communities.

[1] Dwight Longenecker, "Taking The Risk of Faith," *Those Catholic Men*, November 07, 2016, https://thosecatholicmen.com/articles/taking-risk-faith/.

What does it mean to make medical practice an expression of faith? How can manifesting Christian principles through medical practice lead both medical professionals and patients to a greater integration of faith in daily life? By what process can we accomplish this transformation?

To answer these questions, recognize first that refashioning medical practice as a faith-inspired action is not a private activity. It requires us to consider our role in building up Christian communities as fortress and leaven, with an uncompromising adherence to the truth. When we realize that our Christian calling requires us to infuse everything we are and do with the light of faith, we realize that even everyday activities—such as seeking medical care (in the case of patients) or ministering to the sick (in the case of medical professionals)—strengthen relationships of love and draw us closer to God. The actions of seeking or providing medical care are not exempt from our Christian vocation—on the contrary, when performed as acts of faithfulness, they become deep expressions of Christian witness.

Next, seeing medicine as a manifestation of the Christian life requires us to unlearn much of what we have come to assume about how to practice medicine in the present postmodern moment. The dismantling of assumptions opens our minds to escape the confining ideas and presuppositions that the commoditization of medicine has conditioned us to view as indispensable. Such false assumptions have to do with the purported necessity of a litany of regulatory, legislative, financial, and technological innovations upon which modern medicine is said to depend. To let go of these assumptions requires us to reframe our healthcare-related activities (whether as patients or medical professionals) in terms of our Christian vocation, rather than clinging to utilitarian concepts that focus exclusively on efficiency, economics, and data-driven metrics.

Then we ought to learn from other sectors of daily life where redoubled efforts to revive Christian vocation are bearing fruit. Such initiatives provide a model to follow in rebuilding authentically Catholic medicine. One of the most apt parallels for renovating healthcare comes from the field of education. Specifically, the burgeoning Catholic classical K-12 education movement has emerged through the efforts of networks of committed families who have come together to create educational alternatives that provide spiritual and academic nourishment for their children, while also strengthening Christian communities. In a relatively short time, classical Catholic grade schools and high schools have increasingly sprung up across the country. Similarly, in recent years a new cohort of vibrantly Catholic colleges and universities, many of which are recognized by the Cardinal Newman Society, have captured the imagination of faithful Catholic students and families.[2] Their

---

2 For more information, see the Cardinal Newman Society website at https://cardinalnewmansociety.org/college/.

rapidly expanding enrollments and increased public visibility attest to the hunger for formative Catholic higher education.

Now project these educational enterprises' rapid and vigorous success onto a vision for Catholic medicine. Imagine how beautiful it would be for each of these school communities—indeed, for all our parish communities—to be served by a thriving Catholic medical practice, one informed by and adhering to the faith, serving families—domestic churches—across generations!

The Pillars of Catholic Medical Practice

What defines a Christian response to the challenges facing contemporary medicine? How can medical professionals self-assess the system in which they care for patients? How should Christians evaluate the faithfulness of the medical entities where they receive care? If we strive to create medical practices that are consonant with the Catholic social teaching principles already outlined, we must be willing to adhere unconditionally to the truths of our faith. As a foundational example, Christian medicine must always maintain an unwavering dedication to preserving the life and the dignity of the human person, while working to make medical care accessible for all regardless of their place in society. For Christians dedicated to living out the Great Commission through medical care, these principles are nonnegotiable.

Regarding other more prudential matters, such as how to live out this vision for Christian medicine, a faithful approach allows space for medical practices to address local needs in response to conditions on the ground. By appealing to both solidarity and subsidiarity, Christian medical professionals and the communities we serve can retake terrain previously ceded to government, pushing back against the welfare state as we begin to reassert the domain of the Church as the primary organ of ministry. Rather than relying on policy-heavy, top-down solutions to address the needs of the poor through faceless bureaucracies in distant capitals, a properly Christian initiative should reflect the local environment and remain close to people in need. Recentering social responses in the local community rather than relying on public programs may appear paradoxical, because our postmodern, secular age has conditioned us to believe that a more generous welfare state reflects a more compassionate society. Contrary to this belief, remember that we are each expected to practice solidarity as an individual Christian commitment.

For this reason, displacing the responsibility to care for the poor onto faceless bureaucracies does not absolve individual Christians of our duty to tend to the marginalized. And Christians are the very walls of the Church; together we form the mystical Body of Christ. The inherent human dignity that is common to all people is expressed by voluntary works of charity. Such works accentuate the dignity of the giver as well as that of the recipient. As the Catholic professor Anthony Esolen explains, "Catholic social teaching demands full freedom for the Church and for free associations of Christians to do the only real work that can unite rich and poor—and to do so without interference by the State, and without reducing 'welfare' to the mathematical and mechanical definition that is the only one the secular State can give."[3] By relying on expansive governmental social programs to meet basic societal needs, our country has undermined the well of charity present in organic human relationships by which prior generations provided for these needs.

Having applied Catholic social teaching to medicine in broad terms, let us now turn to five pillars of authentic Christian medical practice.

1. A Catholic Healthcare Response Puts Human Dignity at the Center of Its Work Without Compromise

To remain faithful to Christ—who is the Word and Truth itself—we must assent to certain unyielding principles. The greatest of these is the primacy of human dignity as expressed in the theological concept of *imago Dei*. Without an uncompromising commitment to upholding human dignity, the entire Christian medical project is devoid of meaning.

Sadly, the very premise that the Christian physician is free to practice according to the principle of *imago Dei* has been under attack for some time. The liberal secularism that has pervaded Western society dismisses principles that are grounded in transcendental truths. This nihilistic and relativistic worldview has permeated the contemporary medical establishment, leading to the incremental extension of abortion and physician-assisted suicide from merely legalized practices to protected "rights" and newly created standards of care, all while accelerating the erosion of medical professionals' rights of conscience. As Pellegrino argued, "In the past . . . the Hippocratic ethic was the moral *lingua franca* of physicians across history and cultures. Today, consensus on the precepts of the Hippocratic ethic has been seriously eroded. Individual physicians and their professional organizations now hold different positions on the moral status of their relationship with patients. One cannot assume any longer a common formation of professional conscience, or a shared conception of ethical physician behavior."[4]

At the root of mainstream US healthcare's abandonment of Hippocratic principles is a lack of consensus about the primacy of human dignity. This absence is evident when we review the fruits of US healthcare

---

[3] Anthony Esolen, *Reclaiming Catholic Social Teaching: A Defense of the Church's True Teachings on Marriage, Family, and the State* (Sophia Institute Press, 2014), 155.

[4] Pellegrino, *Philosophy of Medicine Reborn*, 288.

reform represented by the passage of the ACA, which continues to shape medical delivery today. As Charles Donovan and Grace-Marie Turner argued in *Linacre Quarterly*, "Neither the system the Affordable Care Act (ACA) reformed, nor the vast scheme of central government mandates and controls that the ACA represents, honored the sanctity of each and every human life and the character of the patient-doctor relationship."[5]

In short, an authentically Christian medical response must safeguard the dignity of human life in all its stages and forms if it is to remain true to its reason for being.

2. *A Catholic Healthcare Enterprise Responds to the Needs of the Poor and Is Offered and Open to All, Regardless of Socioeconomic Status, Race, Religion, or Creed*

In keeping with the principle of solidarity, Christian medicine must do as it has always done: minister to all people, with special attention to those most in need of care. By extending its ministry to include those who are marginalized, Catholic medicine practices what it preaches about the dignity of the human person. Put another way, if medicine exists to serve people—and if each person reflects God's image—then how can we, as people of faith, refuse to serve those made in his image who most need care? When we recognize that the purpose of medicine is to serve people in the light of their inherent human dignity, the Christian healing ministry becomes a way to preach without words by serving as a witness to charity. As St. John Paul II instructed in *Centesimus annus*, "Love for others, and in the first place love for the poor, in whom the Church sees Christ himself, is made concrete in the *promotion of justice*" (emphasis original).[6]

Those who are materially poor often come first to mind when speaking of the marginalized in medicine, but people are afflicted by other forms of lack, or poverty. Referencing the preferential option for the poor, St. John Paul II reminds us that "this option is not limited to material poverty, since it is well known that there are many other forms of poverty, especially in modern society—not only economic but cultural and spiritual poverty as well."[7] By its very nature, medicine ministers

---

[5] Charles A. Donovan and Grace-Marie Turner, "Restoring Christ-Centered Medicine through Public Policy Changes Centered Around Subsidiarity and the Doctor-Patient Relationship," *Linacre Quarterly* 83, no. 4 (November 2016): 387–401, https://doi.org/10.1080/00243639.2016.1254424.

[6] John Paul II, *Centesimus annus*, no. 58, https://www.vatican.va/content/john-paul-ii/en/encyclicals/documents/hf_jp-ii_enc_01051991_centesimus-annus.html.

[7] John Paul II, *Centesimus annus*, no. 57.

to those who suffer from poverty of health; when practiced authentically it cannot help but serve the poor. Recognizing the different forms of poverty that burden those who come for assistance allows us as Christian medical professionals to serve with compassion.

This call for medical ministries to be open to all has another caveat: they must truly be open to everyone, irrespective of race, religion, condition, or station in life. Although secular contemporary ideologies elevate concepts such as inclusion and equity to rectify historical injustices committed against certain demographic categories of people, Christian medical personnel must recognize the humanity in all people who come for care. Because of our call to love unconditionally, Christians must resist the divisiveness of the zeitgeist that serves in fact to dehumanize people by focusing on reductive identities rooted in ethnicity, race, sex, or other characteristics. A worldview that emphasizes such demographic differences to the exclusion of the inherent human dignity of *imago Dei* is, by definition, dehumanizing; and it denies agency to the very people it claims to represent. Such theories' perversion of the concept of dignity is incompatible with a Christian worldview. It certainly has no place in a Christian approach to medical care and should be rejected by the Catholic medical professional.

3. *As a Ministry, Catholic Medical Care Is Rooted in a Local Call to Service Within the Community, in Accordance with the Principle of Subsidiarity*

The principle of subsidiarity, which goes hand in hand with solidarity, opens a space for the grassroots exercise of service that responds intimately to local conditions. Together, subsidiarity and solidarity express people's commitment to respond to the needs of their neighbors. With regard to medicine, this commitment means that the care of the marginalized becomes the responsibility of the Christian. Care for those who are poor and infirm is a personal duty, one that requires a response from individuals; it cannot be relegated to faceless bureaucratic institutions in a faraway capital, legislature, or nongovernmental organization.

Subsidiarity depends on Christian solidarity because people's activities to formulate locally administered responses to community needs would be meaningless without a commitment to the common good that lies at the root of solidarity. Residents' efforts to organize and carry out solutions for local needs highlight their own human dignity, because they recognize their freedom to act in a way that serves God through love of neighbor.

The principle of subsidiarity is undermined by the insidious growth of the belief that all societal problems should be relegated to technocratic systems, such as government. The outsourcing of charity to public welfare programs is damaging for several reasons. First, displacing our personal calling to care for the sick and poor onto bureaucratic entities invites an erroneous sense of complacency on our part—a mistaken belief that we have fulfilled our Christian obligation to the poor. Paying taxes is thus seen as equivalent to private tithing; it absolves us of further burdens of conscience and responsibility. Dependence on public programs to address problems in health care attenuates our culture by making us less charitable. By expanding the welfare regime, ordinary citizens come to assume that material problems have been duly addressed and are no longer their concern. This in turn leads to a callousness of heart, which counteracts the effects of charity.

Finally, overreliance on public programs to provide for healthcare needs is harmful because healthcare-by-committee does a poorer job of addressing needs than the local efforts of engaged citizens. The blunt instruments of legislation, regulation, and funding allocation cannot hold a candle to the labors of people who give of themselves and can respond more effectively and immediately to their neighbors in need. Many who come to rely on public assistance suffer an additional harm: eroding their sense of self-worth by neutralizing their own efforts to provide for themselves and their families. Intergenerational dependence on governmental assistance has a pernicious effect on those whom such assistance purports to help. Chronic recipients of public welfare benefits can come to consider the material benefits of government programs as an entitlement in recompense for their poverty, compensation for which they need not feel any sense of gratitude or obligation in turn to contribute to the common good.

4. Through Conviction to the Gospel, a Truly Medical Witness Remains Independent of the Influences of Public or Corporate Payors That Can Hold Sway over the Way They Carry Out Their Mission of Evangelization and Healing

In the past three-quarters of a century, the practice of medicine has become mired in a tangle of complex regulations and financial encumbrances. The growth of government involvement in healthcare financing and regulation, coupled with the expanding role of health insurers in directing the way medicine is practiced, threatens to strip physicians of our professional autonomy to practice according to our professional expertise and convictions. As a recent example of coercive public policy pitted against rights of conscience, consider the Little Sisters of the Poor order's fourteen-year legal battle against the federal government to seek an exemption from the ACA's contraception mandate.[8] Other legal provisions have contested medical professionals' rights to refuse to participate in abortions, sterilizations, or assisted suicide. Aside from legal imperatives, healthcare professionals are also subject to financial imperatives to engage in practices that violate Christian ethics. Thus, the ideal Christian medical witness must remain distanced from the purse-string influence of these third parties, particularly in areas where government regulations and commercial insurance riddle the delivery system with complexity and sap the vitality from medicine's mission, and where the receipt of public dollars subjects practitioners to governmental violations of conscience.

The need for economic independence from third parties may seem like an impossibility in our highly complex and increasingly costly healthcare system. The idea that any discipline of medicine could develop without the financial support of private insurance companies or governmental payors seems to contradict modern wisdom. Consider the vast differences among medicine's various disciplines. As this book has already pointed out, the technological and staffing expertise needed to run a trauma surgery department is entirely unrelated to the relatively simple operation of an office-based primary care practice. As is always the case when public monies permeate an industry, the accretion of government financing actually causes services' prices to increase relative to the cost of delivering those services. Thus, the goal of establishing a faithfully Christian primary care initiative that is financially free of outside influences represents a more effective form of economic stewardship and is certainly an attainable and laudable pursuit.

Even given the relatively low cost of operating a primary care practice compared to other disciplines within medicine, an office-based practice that declines third-party payment is taking on added financial risk, particularly in a healthcare system that has conditioned patients to depend on insurance for all levels of care. In a primary care clinic that refuses payor contracts, this risk is borne by the physician who founds such a novel practice model. Such physicians are responsible for the practice design and development, for marketing and contracting, and for the provision of patient care. Yet if authentically Christian primary care practices are a communal good, and if such practices help to strengthen families and parishes, such efforts must be able to count on collaboration

[8] See Madalaine Elhabbal, "White House Backs off Contraceptive Mandate, Potential Win for Little Sisters of the Poor," *National Catholic Register*, December 28, 2024, https://www.ncregister.com/cna/white-house-backs-off-contraceptive-mandate-potential-win-for-little-sisters-of-the-poor.

with other areas of the local Christian community that will benefit from this effort. Such support might come from local parishes and churches, faith-based schools, independent businesses, and ordinary citizens who see the value and wish to build up a faith-based health initiative. The cooperation of various segments of the community helps such a practice to fulfill its mission to offer personal, authentically Christian medical care as a form of evangelical witness.

5. Practices That Adhere to Catholic Principles Are Good Stewards of Financial Resources and Human Talents, and They Use These God-Given Gifts to Enhance the Care of Those Whom They Serve

I have already made the case for primary care's proximity and accessibility to ordinary people as a key component to its potency for modeling Christian charity. One other aspect of primary care is its ability to achieve much with little. As much of the rest of medicine relies on increasingly expensive and elaborate technology, primary care can achieve much of its purpose with relatively limited resources.

From a business perspective, maintaining low start-up and operating costs makes good financial sense. The practice becomes economically sustainable more quickly, and it has a higher chance of financial viability than if it required a larger investment in start-up and overhead. However, as already described, the larger purpose of such a practice is to touch lives and minister through corporal works of mercy. A medical practice can reach more people by maximizing the talents and treasure at its disposal. It can also help its patients by simplifying its processes and offering services that improve their ability to adhere to treatment and comply with medical recommendations.

By allotting adequate time for visits, primary care clinicians can address patient concerns more fully. Often this added time means they can also care for a wider scope of issues by offering minor procedures and diagnostic testing that would otherwise be referred to a subspecialist. Such judicious use of time can improve care and increase the clinician's sense of agency in serving patients.

A stewardship-minded practice can further enhance value for patients by contracting certain services to be provided under its roof that might otherwise be sent out. For example, practices that offer phlebotomy in the office and negotiate fees directly with the laboratory add convenience and can save patients sizable amounts of money compared to paying for labs with insurance. Similarly, practices that dispense generic medications at wholesale prices right in the office add value and demonstrate a commitment to prudential stewardship.

Building Benedict Medicine on the Five Pillars

These five pillars provide a blueprint for the basic structure of authentic Christian medical practice in our time. This blueprint relies on a firm foundation of unconditional respect for human dignity. The twin walls of solidarity and subsidiarity are erected on that foundation and in turn hold up a roof that safeguards both the practice and patients from the corrupting influence of external forces, providing shelter for our medical ministry to act according to its mission. The basic outline just described is the outline for what I refer to as Benedict Medicine. In the remaining chapters, I elaborate on the practical application of Benedict Medicine to create a parallel Christian medical witness, starting with the pivotal role played by primary care in its development.

CHAPTER 6

Primary Care as the Beachhead for Implementing Benedict Medicine

"When God created the world He commanded each tree to bear fruit after its kind; and even so He bids Christians, – the living trees of His Church, – to bring forth fruits of devotion, each one according to his kind and vocation."

—St. Francis de Sales[1]

Large-scale changes don't usually happen overnight. Often they come about through a series of smaller, almost imperceptible events. The magnificence of the Grand Canyon today was formed by the slow erosion of the Colorado River over six million years. More than a century and a half passed between the first English colonists' arrival in Jamestown and American independence, which led to the establishment of a new form of citizen self-government. Even our Church's humble beginnings began with Jesus' appointment of a ragtag group of twelve Judean men from different walks of life to the mystical Body of Christ, which now encompasses more than 1.3 billion souls across the globe.[2] Things of marvel do not reach the peak of their splendor in haste. As the saying goes, Rome wasn't built in a day.

In a similar way, the project of reshaping our healthcare system in accordance with Christian principles will not be achieved overnight. It will require discipline, sacrifice, patience, and—above all—the commitment of faith. However, undertaking this endeavor means starting somewhere. And to rebuild authentically Christian medicine, that "somewhere" begins with primary care practices.

---

1 Francis de Sales, *Introduction to the Devout Life*, chap. 3, Christian Classics Ethereal Library, https://ccel.org/ccel/desales/devout_life/devout_life.iii.iii.html.

2 Nina Benedictka Krapic, "Global Catholic Population Rising As Number of Priests, Religious Falls," *Vatican News*, October 20, 2023, https://www.vaticannews.va/en/church/news/2023-10/fides-catholic-church-statistics-world-mission-sunday.html.

Defining Primary Care

What is meant by primary care? When most people hear the term, they think of their family doctor, general internist, or pediatrician. Perhaps it was the doctor they visited with their parents every time they were ill or needed a checkup. Usually, it was the doctor who knew you by name and remembered certain details about your life and your medical history. And nearly always, when you went to that doctor's office, you knew who would be treating you.

Researchers and academics have come up with a more descriptive definition of primary care that echoes many of the qualities I just described. According to researcher Barbara Starfield, effective primary care is characterized by four essential elements: (1) it provides front-line care that is easy to access; (2) it focuses on the person being served, in continuous relationship between the patient and her or his personal doctor; (3) it offers a comprehensive set of services; and (4) it coordinates care when it becomes necessary to refer the patient to a subspecialist.[3]

To Starfield's defining principles of primary care, I add a couple elements. Expanding on her first point, I also note that primary care takes all comers—it does not narrow its scope to a particular disease process, organ system, or patient demographic. Primary care is the discipline within medicine that strives to make sense of the patient's concerns and symptoms *as the patient describes them* and only then comes up with a diagnosis and management plan. Put another way, the primary care physician specializes in the undifferentiated complaint. This approach requires primary care doctors to think more broadly about patient symptoms and histories. A pain in the chest could be related to heart disease, but alternatively it might be due to acid indigestion, asthma, or a pulled muscle. It is the primary doctor's function to combine history taking, physical exam, and clinical experience to determine the best way to diagnose and manage these undifferentiated complaints.

I add another point to Starfield's first and second principles: primary care is best delivered when it is embedded in the community where people live, work, and play. Unlike much subspecialty care provided in hospitals and academic medical centers, primary care is most accessible when it is located in ordinary places close to the people it serves. This proximity makes it easier for people to access their primary care physicians when they need care, which lends itself to my next point.

Here it is: at its heart, primary care is about relationships. Relationships do not magically develop overnight; people need time and repeated encounters to develop bonds of trust. So for people to come to

---

[3] Barbara Starfield, "Family Medicine Should Shape Reform, Not Vice Versa," *Family Practice Management* 16, no. 4 (2009): 6–7.

trust their doctor, it is crucial that they can expect to see their personal physician when they have a health need. Additionally, forging relationships requires time—the secret ingredient and superpower of every great primary care physician.

Primary Care That Bears Christian Witness

These defining characteristics of primary care explain its essential role in establishing a foothold for Christian medical witness to reshape American medicine. By definition, a movement of witness needs to be visible—meaning open and accessible to people from all walks of life. Primary care is an ideal instrument for Christian witness because it is open to care for all people regardless of age, sex, or specific medical condition. It exists within the space where people carry out the business of their daily lives. It requires relatively little in the way of material resources, which means its provision can be adapted for conventional doctor's offices, home visits, medical vans, and even street corners.

Bearing witness is an act of encounter, which also takes time. Under ideal conditions, primary care physicians attend to patients' concerns with the time required to understand their needs. Time allows the doctor to truly know the patient, to consider the cause of the patient's complaint, and to elaborate a detailed management plan. Time also strengthens the doctor-patient bond and assures the patient that his or her concerns are receiving full attention. Most important, the ongoing human relationships that lie at the heart of idealized primary care speak to medicine's transcendent potential and make it the logical linchpin for an effort to renew medical practice as envisioned by Benedict Medicine.

One last advantage that primary care has over subspecialty care in renewing medicine is its economic adaptability. In addition to being geographically and physically accessible, primary care is the least costly care environment in the healthcare system. When it achieves Starfield's four cardinal principles, primary care leads to improved individual and community health, as well as reducing overall healthcare costs.[4]

Factors Impeding Primary Care

Ironically, the legislative and technological solutions that have been introduced over the past few decades—ostensibly to make primary care easier to access—have inflated costs and created unwieldy, impersonal delivery systems. The incremental dependence on health insurance to

---

[4] See Leiyu Shi, "The Impact of Primary Care: A Focused Review," *Scientifica* 2012, https://doi.org/10.6064/2012/432892.

provide access, along with the expansion of governmental programs as a means to make healthcare more affordable—these both have burdened primary care practices with greater regulation and data-reporting requirements that have made it more expensive to provide care. What's more, to meet the demands of third-party payors, practices are forced to design workflows that often make it more difficult for patients to see their personal physician in a timely manner. These same demands shrink the time the primary care physician can dedicate to addressing each patient's needs and concerns, because payor agendas hold doctors accountable for reporting performance data on predetermined care metrics.

Tragically, today's prevailing primary care system does not measure up well with Starfield's principles of ideal primary care. Rather than her personalist approach, contemporary primary care has placed its trust in a systems-based, technological approach. This commoditized system assumes that both patients and clinicians are interchangeable—that is, so long as the number of patients on the schedule matches the number of available appointments, which clinician will see any given patient simply does not matter. Algorithms control everything, from the protocol for scheduling a visit to the management of conditions being scrutinized by data analysts via quality metrics. Insurance companies and government payors determine payment by making convoluted calculations that determine the complexity of the patient's health history, as recorded by clinicians at each visit through standardized diagnostic codes. The promise that enhanced payments will be directed to practices with higher numbers of high-acuity patients give clinicians incentive to make their patients appear as sick as possible through their documentation, in order to increase the "risk adjustment"—a measure of the clinical complexity that estimates the amount of care a particular patient needs.

Primary care delivered through the conventional healthcare system also falls short with respect to the comprehensiveness of care. Oftentimes, the pressure of a heavily booked office schedule means that physicians may not have time to perform procedures or diagnostic interventions for which they have trained. Family physicians, who are trained in residency to care for people of all ages and to perform several office-based procedures, are frequently not given the opportunity to see children or to employ their procedural skills, due to time constraints or other material requirements. When employed by multispecialty groups, primary care physicians are often expected to refer patients to subspecialists to manage conditions that they themselves have been trained to treat. The tensions of time, institutional finances, and departmental politics all play a role in shaping practice patterns to shortchange primary care physicians from offering the breadth of care they are capable of delivering.

Our Glorious Opportunity

Contemporary American primary care thus falls abysmally short of the ideal in our modern healthcare system. Ours is a highly impersonal, fragmented, byzantine system in which primary care physicians often cannot offer the scope of care for which they have prepared. Excessive patient referrals make care coordination more difficult. Insurance policies that require primary care physicians to obtain prior authorization add to practice overhead, increasing the cost of care. Binding patients to doctors via their insurance policies means that changes in insurance can break established therapeutic relationships, while hurried interactions with multiple distractions interfere with building a trusting relationship. Given this dismal scenario, no wonder as much as 64% of primary care physicians reported burnout as recently as 2021.[5]

Ironically, however, this catastrophic situation offers us a glorious opportunity to restore right order to US primary care. By reimagining how primary care medicine can fulfill the larger purpose, or *telos*, of medicine, we can make primary care a highly effective instrument for ministry. By renewing our dedication to preserving life and human flourishing, by making medical care personal and humanistic, by fostering deep relationships between doctors and patients cultivated over time, and by being available to meet as many patients' needs as possible—in all these ways, a revitalized primary care campaign becomes the ideal Christian medical witness.

The threats and barriers to such a renewal of primary care are many. At their root, these obstacles are connected by dependence on the third-party-based system that finances nearly all healthcare today. This same payment system claims the allegiance of well-meaning professionals and practice managers, who must comply with regulatory and data-reporting requirements in order to remain financially solvent. This system is responsible for much of the depersonalization that characterizes contemporary US healthcare.

Recall the story in chapter 1 that described how the University of California voted to end affiliations with Catholic hospitals over their conscientious refusal to cooperate with the evil acts of abortion, direct sterilization, and contraception. That decision is but one example of how hospitals' reliance on public funding subjects them to a mountain of rules and regulations that limit their ability to act according to conscience. Sadly, there are countless examples of Catholic hospitals that

---

[5] Marcus V. Ortega et al., "Patterns in Physician Burnout in a Stable-Linked Cohort," *JAMA Network Open* 6, no. 10 (October 2, 2023), https://doi.org/10.1001/jamanetworkopen.2023.36745.

have been subjected to litigation or financial penalties for simply living out their commitment to uphold the Christian understanding of the human person. Consider another case involving a woman with gender dysphoria, Jesse Hammons, who was scheduled for a hysterectomy as part of a so-called gender-affirming procedure at St. Joseph Medical Center, operated under the auspices of the University of Maryland.[6] When the Catholic hospital, on religious grounds, refused to allow the surgery, the institution was met with a lawsuit launched by the American Civil Liberties Union. Ultimately, the case was decided against St. Joseph's, which was judged to have violated a nondiscrimination clause in the ACA. In the eyes of the law, upholding Catholic anthropology and truth about immutable human sexuality by denying a nontherapeutic surgery is deemed sex discrimination. Such cases illustrate why a Catholic primary care witness can stay fully committed to mission only when it distances itself from anti-Christian policies tied to payments from third parties. When Christian healthcare entities get snared in these legal bear traps, their healing ministries are drained of essential resources, and the spiritual aspect of their mission comes under siege. Christian hospital systems and other more complex areas of care delivery are particularly threatened in this way because often they depend on government funding to operate. In contrast, Christian primary care efforts are nimbler and better able to focus on the personal aspect of their ministry by remaining free of the entanglements that are part and parcel with insurance and government contracting.

Where can we find tangible models of the practical application of Benedict Medicine in primary care? What examples today can inform a Christian primary care witness? I explore some answers in chapter 7.

---

[6] Brooke Migdon, "Maryland Hospital Violated Affordable Care Act in Denying Medical Care to Trans Patient, Court Rules," *The Hill*, January 6, 2023, https://thehill.com/regulation/court-battles/3803034-maryland-hospital-violated-affordable-care-act-in-denying-medical-care-to-trans-patient-court-rules/.

CHAPTER 7

Examples from Our Time: Learning from What Exists

"An adventure is only an inconvenience rightly considered. An inconvenience is only an adventure wrongly considered."

—G. K. Chesterton[1]

Chapter 6 made the case for why primary care is the proper venue to spearhead the renewal of medicine; I concluded with a promise to provide examples to guide this project. Fortunately several exemplary models can serve as an invaluable source of inspiration and hope for the development of Benedict Medicine. To imagine their implications for authentically Christian primary care offers nothing if not an adventure, as this chapter will show.

In *The Seven Habits of Highly Effective People*, businessman Stephen Covey speaks of the dual process inherent in the creative process: that all things are first visualized in the mind before they are physically created.[2] Applying Covey's aphorism to Christian medical witness, to make tangible the project of Benedict Medicine, we must first imagine how such practices are embodied and exist in the real world. The best way to envision such a reality is by studying examples of how real people in real communities are already applying Christian principles to medical care.

The Purpose of the Practice

Let's remind ourselves of the overarching purpose, or *telos*, of the practice of medicine. As earlier chapters examined, the profession exists in service to those who are sick: to alleviate suffering, restore health, and promote human flourishing. Bioethicists Farr Curlin and Christopher Tollefsen

1 G. K. Chesterton, *On Running After One's Hat and Other Whimsies* (Robert M. McBride & Company, 1933), 6, https://archive.org/details/onrunningafteron027309mbp/page/n17/mode/2up.

2 Stephen R. Covey, *The Seven Habits of Highly Effective People*, rev. ed. (Simon & Schuster, 2020), 113.

remind us that "medicine is a paradigmatic practice, elevated to a profession because of its social importance, that aims at human health."[3] By implication, any activity that works against the betterment of human health thereby contravenes the social covenant of the medical profession.

At its core, medicine is about service. The primary object of this service is the patient who presents for care. Medicine without a patient is somewhat like a soccer match without a ball, in that it lacks the object which gives it purpose. The patient seeks either the alleviation of suffering or restoration of health in some capacity; the patient comes because he or she has a need that requires attention. However, when service through medicine is considered in broader terms, its ripples extend well beyond the individual patient who passes through the clinic door. As with other forms of Christian service, the healing profession also bestows graces on those who serve—it gives their lifelong commitment and their daily work a deep sense of meaning and purpose. That meaning is the taproot of compassion, and helps professionals to remain strong while witnessing enormous suffering. Tragically, today's commoditized third-party payor model of healthcare has devalued the dedication and agency of the medical professionals who are its most valuable and irreplaceable assets. The diminishment of their commitment is, in my view, the greatest contributor to the epidemic of burnout among healthcare workers that has smoldered unabated for several years.

While the profession of medicine serves patients and gives purpose to the work of clinicians, its positive effects ripple even further into the broader community. When medicine improves individuals' health, the gains spill over and multiply benefits to others who live and work alongside those individuals. By adding the spiritual conviction of medicine practiced by clinicians of faith as an act of charity, in concordance with the principles of Benedict Medicine, this ripple effect has the potential to expand into a transformative tidal wave of evangelization by example.

What Does Benedict Medicine Look Like in Practice?

We can preview the practical outpouring of grace of the Benedict Medicine approach by focusing on just a few of the many concrete examples of charity through healthcare. Let's begin with an example of Christian solidarity that, while not directly clinical, offers insight and inspiration into building up a healing Christian community through mutual aid.

The Christian practice of coming together to pool resources and support one another in difficult times has existed since the early Church. In

[3] Farr Curlin and Christopher Tollefsen, *The Way of Medicine: Ethics and the Healing Profession* (University of Notre Dame Press, 2021), 4.

the United States, Amish and Mennonite communities have relied on this practice for centuries.[4] In the late twentieth century, a formalized approach to healthcare cost-sharing expanded to several other Christian communities and began to serve as an insurance alternative for meeting the medical needs of families. In cost-sharing ministries, participating individuals and families contribute monthly tithes to the ministry, funds that are then used to help members who have outstanding medical bills. The organizing entity negotiates prices with medical service providers on behalf of its members. In this sense, health share ministries are not insurance—they do not create coverage contracts for specific services, and members pay doctors directly and are not restricted to provider networks, as is the case with healthcare insurance.

Health share ministries exemplify the principle of solidarity by bringing together the contributions of Christians to serve the common good. Empowering individuals to decide where they receive care honors the concept of subsidiarity by relegating these intimate decisions to the level of the family. Health share ministries sidestep the intermediaries and inflated costs associated with insurance, while also contributing to good stewardship of resources. They offer one key model for how Benedict Medicine can put Catholic social teaching into practice.

Catholic Social Teaching in Practice

One seminal example of a primary care practice founded on the principles of Catholic social teaching is St. Luke's Family Practice in Modesto, California. The result of the inspirational vision of Robert Forrester, St. Luke's was designed to address the care needs of the broader community, including local agricultural workers who lack access to care. The pro bono care St. Luke's offers the uninsured is made possible through the financial support of more affluent patients, known as benefactors, who pay an annual fee in return for same-day visits and 24/7 physician access. The practice does not contract with insurers or government programs, and half of its clinical care serves the uninsured in the community. With an initial board of directors comprising parishioners and religious from Forrester's parish, St. Luke's is the first medical office in the country to have qualified for 501(c)(3) tax-exempt status as a nonprofit.[5]

While "concierge" practices typically charge retainer fees in addition to billing insurance for affluent patients in return for added services, St.

---

[4] Gari-Anne Patzwald and William Kostlevy, "From Mutual Aid to Global Action," *Christian History*, no. 84 (2004), https://christianhistoryinstitute.org/magazine/article/from-mutual-aid-to-global-action.

[5] Robert A. Forrester, "A New Model of Charitable Care: The Robin Hood Practice," *Family Practice Management* 15, no. 2, (February 2008): 12–16.

Luke's Family Practice marries personalized care for benefactor-patients with expanded care for the area's migrant farmworkers. St. Luke's story exemplifies solidarity with the poor through its clinical care and through the financial support provided by community members with greater means. The practice's initial blueprint and its implementation developed through the prayerful discernment of Forrester and his partner, Richard Heck, and through the dedication of fellow parishioners who formed the initial board of directors. Thus, the creation of St. Luke's Family Practice represents a local solution to a critical need to deliver responsive primary medical care to the area's large population of uninsured—mostly agricultural laborers and their families.[6]

Incorporating the Mission of Catholic Social Teaching

A practice's adherence to Catholic social teaching does not depend on its business structure. Homestead Direct Primary Care (DPC) in Colorado Springs, Colorado, is an example of a practice incorporated as a for-profit business that nonetheless exemplifies stewardship, subsidiarity, and respect for the dignity of the human person. The practice's founder and practicing physician, Rachel Langley, started the practice in August 2023 after being laid off from her former practice. The experience of being let go allowed her to better listen to God's voice calling her to start her own practice.[7]

A distinguishing feature of Homestead DPC is its vibrant activity in the community. Langley is a frequent speaker at local community events, such as parenting groups and social venues for veterans (Langley herself is a former active-duty member of the Air Force and is still an Air Force reservist). She staffs a first aid booth at an annual local parade and festival every August. Her practice attracts young families, who are drawn to her experience as a lactation consultant and leader in La Leche League and her training in the NaProTECHNOLOGY method of natural family planning—she is the only doctor in town with this training. Her community outreach extends to offering care through the local food bank, providing samples of pediatric medications to the local crisis pregnancy house, and hosting medical students for rotations in the practice throughout the year.

[6] For more information, see the St. Luke's Family Practice website: https://stlukesfp.org/.

[7] The information in this section is courtesy of Rachel Langley, personal communication, February 25, 2025.

Through the work of Homestead DPC, Langley has also served her diocese by working with local natural family planning teachers and with the diocesan office of family life. She speaks at parish forums on topics of interest to the lay faithful. The bishop blessed her medical practice's office when it opened and has continued to recognize its contributions.

As the name suggests, Homestead DPC operates on an economic model that provides care to patients for a monthly subscription fee. The practice attracts patients from different ages and stages of life; its lack of reliance on insurance contracts means it does not exclude patients because of insurance status. Homestead DPC's integration into the social fabric of Colorado Springs builds solidarity with individual residents and with community organizations that also work for the common good. The local emphasis and financial independence of Homestead DPC allow it to respond to community needs and promote responsible stewardship for the families it serves.

Institutional Partnerships to Create Benedict Medicine

The story of Gianna Family Care in Shawnee, Kansas, is an inspirational reminder of the key role of institutional support in creating space for Catholic primary care. The practice's founder, family physician Angeliqué Pritchett, had been dissatisfied with the nature of employed corporate practice. Knowing of her discontent, a nurse in her former practice called the Archdiocese of Kansas City, Kansas, to find out if the staff knew of more suitable practice opportunities for Pritchett. The nurse's call coincided with a letter sent to the archbishop from the National Gianna Center—a pro-life medical practice in New York—seeking an entrepreneurial, pro-life physician who might be interested in forming a Gianna Center affiliate in the greater Kansas City area. When Pritchett caught wind of this inquiry, she was sold on the idea. Thus, Gianna Family Care was born.[8]

Like Homestead DPC, Gianna Family Care serves patients according to the model of direct primary care. The practice's operation relies on monthly subscriptions paid by patients, not on insurance or public payors—allowing the practice to maintain its focus on patient care in accordance with Catholic teaching. Among the populations it serves are members of health share ministries, those dissatisfied with the impersonal nature of corporate medical practice structures, and families seeking care that affirms Catholic teaching on procreation. The practice's two physicians are trained in NaProTECHNOLOGY, the natural family

[8] The information in this section is courtesy of Angeliqué Pritchett, personal communication, March 28, 2025.

planning method that can also support treatment of infertility, high-risk pregnancies, and gynecological disorders. The practice serves adults and children in the office, and its services include obstetrical care and newborn hospital care.

Since opening in 2016, Gianna Family Care has developed a close collaboration with the archdiocese. Gianna Family Care provides care to archdiocesan employees and their spouses, which the archdiocese subsidizes as part of its health insurance benefits options. This relationship has enabled Gianna Family Care to grow steadily while offering an independent primary care option in accordance with Catholic teaching that supports the archdiocese and the people to whom it ministers. The cooperation affords the archdiocese, in return, access to ethically aligned, broad-scope primary care for a fixed cost for its employees, reducing unnecessary and costly emergency room and urgent-care visits. More importantly, archdiocesan support has made possible this partnership with a medical practice that reflects its evangelical mission.

Responding to the Needs of the Poor and the Immigrant

Another primary care clinic that responds to the needs of the poor out of Christian charity is Clínica Médica Moscati in Huntsville, Alabama. The clinic opened in October 2020, in the throes of the COVID-19 pandemic. But as executive director Mayra Short tells it, the genesis of the idea came years earlier, when she first visited a migrant work camp and felt called to serve those who were poor and far from their homelands. She and her husband Tom, a physician and the medical director of the clinic, decided to open a primary medical clinic to cater to the needs of Hispanic/Latino workers, many of whom were undocumented. As they recount, the Holy Spirit was visibly at work in the clinic's formation. Short created the clinic's 501(c)(3) paperwork online, and within three days a bilingual nurse practitioner wanted to work with them. When they could not find space for lease online, they began to drive around Huntsville looking for a space to open their clinic. They came upon an office in the medical district with a "for rent" sign and met with the owner. As Short tells it, she was a bit sheepish when the woman asked about the plans for the practice. "We are going to open a Catholic medical practice to serve undocumented Hispanic farm workers," she explained. To her surprise, the owner exclaimed that she was a fellow parishioner in their church, and she offered the Shorts the office at a reduced rent.[9]

---

[9] The information in this section is courtesy of Mayra Short, personal communication, February 14, 2025.

The clinic offers the full-time care of a nurse practitioner, as well as separate subspecialty services from volunteer physicians in internal medicine, rheumatology, gastroenterology, endocrinology, and urology. The practice uses paper charts, avoiding more expensive electronic medical records to save money. Patients, who are mostly Hispanic/Latino agricultural workers, are asked to make a modest payment per visit, although the practice does not turn away people who are unable to pay. However, patient fees do not cover the clinic's expenses; additional grant money and donations cover the remaining operational costs, although Short recalls that the clinic's budget was deep in the red in the early years. "For the first two years we were sweating bullets," she recounts. Over time, though, generous grants from the local hospital foundation, the local chapter of the St. Vincent de Paul Society, and others have filled the gap, demonstrating to the Shorts that the Lord provides what is needed at the right time.

Since opening Clínica Médica Moscati, Mayra and Tom Short have made it clear to all that the clinic exists to serve the Lord. Images of St. Guiseppe Moscati (the clinic's patron), Our Lady of Guadalupe, and the Sacred Heart of Jesus greet patients and visitors. Mayra Short describes several instances when visitors and benefactors shared their own observations of the clinic's tangible faith witness. Many of the clinic's collaborating volunteer physicians, community members, and patients do not share the Shorts' Catholic faith, yet they still contribute their time, talent, and treasure to further its mission. Short sees the support of the larger community as a message for Christian medicine: "the Lord is going to send you people of good will."

Clínica Médica Moscati does not contract with insurance companies, Medicare, or Medicaid—concerned that third-party payments come with strings attached that could compromise the clinic's unapologetic Catholic witness. Short says, "People are hungry to see the faith being lived with boldness. As Jesus teaches, we cannot light a lamp and set it under a bushel basket." She says the Lord is allowing the clinic to continue because its witness is needed. As an example of that witness, she recalls a young woman suffering with advanced rheumatoid arthritis, who labors in construction to make a living despite the pain and deformity of her arthritis-stricken hands. Service to the poor who would otherwise go without care is the mission of Clínica Médica Moscati, serving as an example of solidarity, subsidiarity, and stewardship in a nonprofit model.[10]

---

[10] Mayra Short, personal communication, February 14, 2025.

✠

The preceding five examples of Christian witness in medicine demonstrate very different approaches to proclaiming the transcendentally spiritual dimension of medical care. What unifies them as examples of Catholic social teaching in action is their simplicity and conformity with the principles of the defense of human dignity, solidarity, subsidiarity, and faithful stewardship. All four originate in a local response to a social need: the need for accessible, comprehensive medical care at the community level. Each addresses this need in a manner that reflects its individual strengths and talents, with a unique focus that responds to that need in a personal way. By organizing personal and local resources to resolve this need, the organizers of these healthcare ministries act in accordance with the principles of distributism, an economic theory that reflects a local and practical application of Catholic social teaching at work in the world. One such distributist idea, summed up by the phrase "three acres and a cow," states that the means of production are best left to private ownership, so that individuals and families can subsist on the honest fruits of their daily work.[11] This aphorism reflects distributism's agrarian origins to make the point that people ought to be able to make a living and support a family from the dignified work using their own resources. When the principle is applied to medicine, clinicians' ability to provide care within their communities, either as individuals or as locally organized groups, conforms to this idea of self-determination and ownership of one's skills, applied for the common good. A distributist approach to medicine stands in stark contrast to the prevailing medical paradigm, in which venture capital–owned practices and health systems employ a larger share of clinicians, thus hamstringing their clinical agency and directing their energies to further corporate goals, which often run counter to the ideals of the Hippocratic profession.

Another important parallel among these healthcare enterprises is that they recognize and lead with their spiritual purpose—that is, to exhibit charity through their actions. Their profession of faith is not incidental to their activities; rather, faith is central to their mission and informs their every action and decision. Thus, whether a health share organizes Christian mutual aid or a primary care practice cares for people's medical needs, such organizations seek to extend Christian charity and reflect Christ's healing mission through their daily work.

One final commonality among the organizations highlighted in this chapter is their intentional effort to safeguard individual rights of

[11] Thomas Storck, "Distributism?—or, Three Acres and a Cow?" *The Chesterton Review* 44, nos. 1/2 (Spring/Summer 2018): 77–87, https://doi.org/10.5840/chesterton2018441/212.

conscience and maintain effective stewardship of the resources of the practices and of the people they serve. By relinquishing the financial advantages of insurance contracts and public assistance programs, these groups maintain control over their clinical and business decisions. They maintain associations and partnerships that align with their missions while disregarding the directives of third-party payors that might compromise their integrity as medical and spiritual enterprises. The absence of outside payors, while creating a relative financial hardship for these practices, paradoxically creates a greater degree of solidarity and subsidiarity as they strengthen local relationships and come to rely on patients and community organizations to serve and grow.

Studying organizations that manifest the principles of Benedict Medicine moves these ideas from abstract concepts to concrete examples. But these are only a handful of ways in which individuals have brought these principles to life. The next chapter considers a broader range of ways for practices to live out the Catholic social principles of Benedict Medicine.

CHAPTER 8

What Does Benedict Medicine Look Like? Practical Aspects

"The simplification of anything is always sensational."

- G. K. Chesterton[1]

What distinguishes a Benedict Medicine practice based in Catholic social teaching? What does it look like? How do patients know when they have found one? This chapter looks at the hallmarks of Christian primary care so that physicians who wish to practice this way will have a lodestar at the start of their journey. Laypeople searching for such a medical practice can also know when they've found one based on the information in this chapter.

I approach this task by returning to the five pillars from chapter 5, with the goal of considering how medical practices can incorporate these principles. One defining characteristic of such practices is their reliance on design simplicity—removing the complexity and cacophony of the modern secular healthcare infrastructure to allow greater focus on a mission of connection and healing.

First, I want to clarify that this chapter offers an overarching approach to discerning or developing a medical practice that adheres to Catholic social teaching and Christian witness. It is not meant to be prescriptive; similarly, it does not imply that Christians of goodwill may not respond to the commitment of faith in ways that differ from this approach. The Christian life is challenging, and the Lord charges each person to fulfill this commitment according to his or her unique calling. Having said this, I offer the following points with humility and in the hope that they will serve as a guide and inspiration for medical professionals and laypeople alike. Each pillar includes reflection questions to guide thinking and assessment. Let us look at the practical applications of the five pillars of Benedict Medicine.

---

[1] G. K. Chesterton, in *The Quotable Chesterton*, ed. Kevin Belmonte (Thomas Nelson, 2011), Kindle.

1. A Catholic Healthcare Response Puts Human Dignity at the Center of Its Work Without Compromise

The Benedict Medicine practice understands that human dignity derives from the human person's creation in the image and likeness of God. This understanding is evident in the way that patients, visitors, and staff are treated. The treatment of all people by such physicians exemplifies St. John Paul II's teaching on human dignity: "God has imprinted his own image and likeness on man (cf. Gen 1:26), conferring upon him an incomparable dignity. . . . In effect, beyond the rights which man acquires by his own work, there exist rights which do not correspond to any work he performs, but which flow from his essential dignity as a person."[2]

Benedict Medicine practices offer care that mirrors this belief in *imago Dei* by asserting the essential dignity of all persons regardless of their state, station, or phase of development. Practices that affirm this truth promote authentic human flourishing. A physician dedicated to safeguarding life neither engages in nor refers for procedures that detract from the dignity of the human person, properly understood, whether the person is in the earliest stages of life or at life's end. Such a physician regards her or his Christian commitment and solemn oath as preeminent in determining her or his conduct, which does not depend on whether a particular practice or protocol is protected by law. For this reason, the Benedict Medicine physician does not compromise when asked to participate or be complicit in acts that destroy, manufacture, or prevent the development of human life at either end of the lifespan. Such a physician acknowledges his or her accountability to God as the primary Judge, who gives rise to the desire for virtuous practice.

Respect for human dignity also manifests itself in the way such a practitioner approaches the care for people with various limitations and disabilities. Whether patients' infirmities are cognitive, physical, developmental, or spiritual, the medical practitioner who respects human dignity seeks to meet the needs of everyone who comes for care by striving to restore bodily functioning and order and to promote consonance of body, mind, and soul. In some cases, this respect for authentic dignity means telling the patient inconvenient truths with gentle clarity and charity. The word "doctor" derives from the Latin *docere*, meaning "to teach." Modern doctors draw from this origin of their title when they explain the truth about patients' conditions and possible remedies. Accepting false premises and sidestepping the truth are incompatible with faithful medical practice and should be identified and avoided to support true human dignity.

[2] John Paul II, *Centesimus annus*, no. 11.

A caveat to this discussion of human dignity is that authentic Benedict Medicine practitioners avoid leading patients astray by aiding or condoning truly immoral acts. Counseling, prescribing, or otherwise sanctioning interventions, prescribed substances, or behaviors that denigrate human dignity or lead to objectively sinful behavior jeopardize the physical and spiritual well-being of the patient; both the physician and the practice commit scandal, which the *Catechism* defines as "an attitude or behavior which leads another to do evil."[3] Aside from commonly cited actions that destroy human life (e.g., abortion, physician-assisted suicide, in vitro fertilization), certain "harm reduction" practices can also undermine human dignity. An example is the prescription of pre-exposure prophylaxis to reduce the risk of contracting HIV during premeditated promiscuous sexual activity (so-called disco dosing). Such prescribing practices promote the assumption that the patient with a penchant for sexual promiscuity is incapable of remaining sexually continent, is at heightened risk for sexually transmitted infections, and thereby requires a technological solution in the form of prophylactic pharmaceuticals. When patients present with such requests, they must be met with compassion and encouragement in a way that does not comply with acts that harm them physically and spiritually.

For reflection: How does the medical practice reflect an authentic Christian vision of the human person? Does it offer care that promotes human flourishing at all phases and stages of life?

2. *A Catholic Healthcare Enterprise Responds to the Needs of the Poor and Is Offered and Open to All, Regardless of Socioeconomic Status, Race, Religion, or Creed*

In keeping with the first pillar, the defense of human dignity also presupposes a desire to serve the common good in solidarity. A Christian medical practitioner is aware of this special duty to those on the margins—the materially poor, as well as people who lack other resources to engage in proper medical care. By considering ways to open his or her practice to people from varying economic levels and medical needs, the faithful physician honors the dignity of all and helps the practice to embody the Christian response that counters the impersonal nature of the public welfare state. When individuals take on the responsibility to shoulder others' burdens and treat them with love and care, the effects are magnified and extend well beyond the individuals being served. Such care softens the hearts of so many others who will see this form of care as witnessing to a much greater force, one that has the capacity to

[3] *Catechism of the Catholic Church,* no. 1883.

change the course of history. Recall from chapter 1 the experience of the Christian healers during the Plague of Cyprian in the 250s AD.

While the ethos of solidarity and service of the common good is common to all practices following Benedict Medicine, the unique gifts and circumstances of each physician and practice naturally lend themselves to more focused emphases. Each of us is endowed with different gifts, just as St. Paul tells us when he says that the members of the Church are like different parts of the same body (see 1 Corinthians 12). As described in the previous chapter, practices such as Clínica Médica Moscati concentrate their efforts on service to undocumented Hispanic/Latino laborers, while other practices highlight care for children, young families, or those confined to the house or nursing facility. Each practice reflects a particular charism for service that the Lord has given to those entrusted with that practice's founding and development. Although each practice may differ in emphasis, all Benedict Medicine practices convey a disposition to serve vulnerable people through their work.

While all medical practices can be said (rightly) to serve the poor because sickness represents an impoverishment of health, practices in the mold of Benedict Medicine see their care as part of a larger effort to tend to people's physical bodies in ways that also account for the preservation of their souls. The act of caring for the sick takes on a more profound spiritual meaning when one carries out that daily care as an expression of the corporal acts of mercy.

For reflection: How does the practice manifest the principle of Christian solidarity? Does it offer care for the poor and marginalized in its treatment of those who are materially poor, spiritually poor, or defenseless?

3. *Catholic Medical Ministry Is Rooted in a Local Call to Service Within the Community, in Accordance with the Principle of Subsidiarity*

Practices that engage in Benedict Medicine respond to a local call to serve a need within their communities. They are intimately familiar with those needs because they too are members of the communities where they practice. This familiarity informs their decisions about how best to address local problems and respond to community-level concerns.

Practices designed to recognize the principle of subsidiarity rely on the engagement of other people and organizations around them for support and guidance. Partnership with others expresses a solidarity that also builds up the local community in ways that are not possible in isolation. Recalling the distributists' "three acres and a cow" idea described in chapter 7, subsidiarity also means that practitioners in independent practice should be able to provide for their own families through their work, analogous to rural landowners who till their own plots to meet their domestic needs. This approach contrasts greatly with the increasing loss of clinical and financial agency over the practice of medicine that medical professionals experience when they are employed by large and impersonal healthcare corporations that often span large geographic areas.

For reflection: Is the practice locally owned and operated? Does it represent a local response to the needs of the community? Does it integrate its work with other local groups and organizations?

4. A Truly Gospel-Focused Medical Witness Remains Independent of the Influences of Public or Corporate Payors

The truly independent, ministry-focused medical practice limits engagement with outside influences that can influence the way it carries out its mission. As discussed elsewhere in this book, US healthcare is driven largely by regulations imposed by agencies such as CMS, with private insurers following suit. When healthcare service providers are attached to third parties by the purse strings, they become de facto bound by the rules created by those entities and approved by CMS. In many cases, the cost of complying with such regulations takes resources away from providing care; in other instances, such directives directly oppose Christian anthropology and fly in the face of Benedict Medicine principles.

Again, financial structure, as an example of subsidiarity, requires a nuanced individual approach, recognizing that different practices must choose different approaches in accordance with local conditions. Still, reliance on third-party payors leaves faithful medical practices vulnerable to the directives of government and corporations. For those primary care practices that wish to remain free from the encumbrances of third parties, a few plausible options exist.

The first option is to seek contributions from other people and entities of goodwill who support the practice's mission. This funding can be solicited by fundraising, applying for grants (for those incorporated as nonprofits), or taking other actions such as crowdfunding. Another benefit of such strategies is the "proof of concept" that comes from developing successful fundraising campaigns among supporters who value the fruits of the practice's mission and wish to contribute to its success.

A second way for practices to remain independent of third-party financial constraints is to seek direct support from those they serve in their daily work. Recent years have brought a groundswell of practices in models termed "direct primary care," which offer primary care services for a flat monthly fee paid by the patient. Far from being elitist or out of touch, these direct primary care practices often serve everyday people who are attracted to their mission and added value. Contrary to accusations of exclusivity, such practices are particularly valuable for people who are uninsured or underinsured and have chronic health conditions that require ongoing monitoring and management by a physician who offers comprehensive primary care. In many respects, direct primary care practices can be thought of as a form of medical cooperative that is supported by the monthly contributions of those they serve. This localist concept harkens, again, to the distributist approach discussed in the third pillar.

For reflection: Does the practice's business structure reduce its susceptibility to coercion from outside forces? What safeguards does it implement to protect its essential mission as a Christ-centered enterprise?

5. *Practices That Adhere to Catholic Principles Are Good Stewards of Financial Resources and Human Talents to Enhance Care*

Continuing the theme of pillar four, the prudent stewardship of resources is a hallmark of the Benedict Medicine practice. By directing financial resources wisely, combined with effective time management and the proper use of the talents of practitioners and staff, Benedict Medicine practices exercise efficacious stewardship that allows their work to be more fruitful and to benefit more people.

Resource stewardship to enhance quality and scope of care is a virtuous practice that serves justice and the common good. Examples of good stewardship include practices' decisions to negotiate the costs of certain ancillary services, such as laboratory and imaging studies, with those service providers in order to make them available to patients at lower cost. When such laboratory contracting also allows labs to be drawn in the office, the convenience for patients also represents effective stewardship of patients' time.

Speaking of time, remember that time spent cultivating relationships is an essential resource for the mission of a Benedict Medicine practice, a resource with no substitutes. Whether physicians take extra time with a patient during a clinical encounter, spend time with clinic staff, or share their time with community members who may be intrigued by the distinctive nature of a Christian practice, investing one's time in and with others is ultimately what the personal calling of medicine is all about. In my own experience, the greatest riches yielded from this investment are the human connection and trust that are strengthened in the process. The doctor-patient relationship, developed on mutual trust over time, fulfills the healing nature of primary care.

For reflection: **What are the practice's greatest resources? How does it invest those resources to achieve its purpose? How does this call to stewardship affect the way it serves patients?**

Summary

Practices can live out the principles of the five pillars in ways that vary almost as much as the number of practices themselves. Rather than narrowing a restrictive list of features or structures, Benedict Medicine is about considering how practices live out Catholic social principles through their work. The simplicity in the way they carry out their mission is a key element in their ability to remain focused on care for the patient as an expression of Christian charity. In the final chapter, I elaborate on some action items for both medical practitioners and faithful laypeople who wish to promote the concepts of Benedict Medicine in their own families and communities.

CHAPTER 9

A Call to Action and Evangelization: How You Can Bring About Benedict Medicine

"Let us get up then, at long last, for the Scriptures rouse us when they say: It is high time for us to arise from sleep *(Rom 13:11). Let us open our eyes to the light that comes from God, and our ears to the voice from heaven that every day calls out this charge:* If you hear his voice today, do not harden your hearts *(Ps 94[95]:8)."*

—St. Benedict of Nursia[1]

We've now arrived at the culmination of this book—the practical application of the principles of Benedict Medicine already discussed. For both medical professionals and individuals seeking this approach to medical care, the hardest question is where to start. For people who would like to encounter a primary care practice with these characteristics, give thorough attention to how a practice addresses the reflection questions of the five pillars (chapter 8) as a useful guide about whether a practice truly represents these principles. For physicians who desire to practice in a way that more fully responds to their faith commitment, reflecting on the answers to those same questions is a reliable compass.

The ideas I put forth in this chapter are largely derived from my own firsthand experience in developing and launching a Christ-centered family practice at the same time I was writing this book. The process of developing the practice offers daily lessons about the challenges and joys of striving to consecrate one's professional identity and purpose to be directed by and to serve the Lord. This experience of relying on others for advice, reassurance, and support reaffirms the idea that as Christians we are called to live in community. Without the assistance and encouragement of those around us, we can begin to doubt in the efficacy of our work, and that doubt mutes its effectiveness. Most of all, this work

[1] Benedict of Nursia, Prologue, in *The Rule of St. Benedict in English*, ed. Timothy Fry (Liturgical Press, 2019). Emphasis original.

underscores the need for absolute humility and reliance on God. The degree of success or failure of our worldly endeavors depends entirely on his providence and our openness to hear his call. He has surprises in store for each of us, if we only allow him into our trials!

Everything Worthwhile Begins with Prayer

Amid major life decisions and challenges, we find it easy to get distracted from the essential and often simple things that should go without saying. One need, frequently overlooked in such circumstances, is the need for prayer. A book about applying Christian principles in medicine would be negligent if it did not emphasize prayerful reflection in this process.

For physicians contemplating a major change in the way we practice, regular prayer is an essential component of this discernment. The decision to adopt a different, countercultural approach to practicing medicine by offering it up in service to the Lord is challenging and invites uncertainty. Considering this uncertainty can in turn provoke fear and anxiety. Reorienting our professional lives according to spiritual pursuits is not like other professional calculations with which we are more familiar. This reorientation involves something much greater, something transcendental. It is not amenable to being deliberated on a notepad with "pro" and "con" columns in the way we might make other decisions about where to study or what house to live in.

Prayerful discernment is critical to this decision and reorientation because it forces us to recognize humbly that the outcome does not depend on our efforts. Rather, we must submit ourselves and our desire to be in control to the force of the Holy Spirit, who will likely take us along paths we did not anticipate or did not wish to travel. For most physicians, this submission runs counter to the type A personality, by which many of us have attributed professional success to a sense of personal control.

In contrast, transforming our practice of medicine in conformity with the principles of Benedict Medicine requires that we be open to daily surprises. We must remember that we will have days—even weeks—of desolation, and that these will be interspersed with moments of consolation. We must cling to those moments of reprieve and imbibe from the springs of hope to rejuvenate our spirits when the Lord graces us with his consolation. The words of St. John Henry Newman can offer us further solace:

> God has created me to do Him some definite service. He has committed some work to me which He has not committed to another. . . . I shall do good; I shall do His work; I shall be

> an angel of peace, a preacher of truth in my own place, while not intending it, if I do but keep His commandments and serve Him in my calling. Therefore, I will trust Him. Whatever, wherever I am, I can never be thrown away. . . . He may take away my friends; He may throw me among strangers, He may make me feel desolate, make my spirits sink, hide the future from me—still He knows what He is about.[2]

Mission Territory

For clinicians embarking on the path to a faith-centered practice—and for those who support such practices by entrusting them with your health and financial support—realize that you are truly entering mission territory. Secular culture and conventional medicine do not have the vocabulary to convey the significance of this form of practice. People in the prevailing system will not always know how to react to the message you transmit through your dedicated efforts. Their lack of understanding will test your efforts in ways with which you may not be familiar. This adversity is to be expected. It comes with being a medical missionary in your own backyard.

Maintaining an active daily prayer life and regular participation in the sacraments is another essential part of remaining spiritually grounded and growing in faith while you redirect your professional activities toward God. If you feel stuck in a spiritual desert, take this time to explore other forms of prayer that enliven your faith. Regularly spend an hour (or more) with the Blessed Sacrament in your parish or a nearby adoration chapel. Offer to the Lord your spiritual dryness—those times when you lack devotion or consolation—as well as your insecurities, doubts, and fears. Place them at the foot of the Cross, where he can direct your thoughts and actions according to his holy will. Study the lives of the saints, particularly those blessed with a charism for healing. Recall the trials that confronted those faced with spiritual desolation, and pray for their intercession and guidance when you face your own difficult moments.

Another response to the spiritual challenges that will surely come is to seek out a spiritual adviser if you do not already have one. Seeking prayerful guidance from someone experienced in the faith and trained to help advisees grow closer to God is a powerful step toward discernment through a time of intense challenge and change. Unlike family, friends, and colleagues who may have other vested (albeit well-intentioned)

---

[2] John Henry Newman, *Meditations and Devotions of the Late Cardinal Newman* (Longmans, Green and Co., 1908), 301, https://www.newmanreader.org/works/meditations/meditations9.html#doctrine1.

interests, a spiritual director is motivated only to help an advisee hear the Lord's voice and answer his call.

Initial Steps Toward a Benedict Medicine Practice

Benedict Medicine medical care offers as many origin stories as there are practices. Often, the movements of the heart stir a single physician to contemplate shifting to an integrated practice and spiritual life. In other cases, a small contingent of individuals in the community come together to start an organization dedicated to service through healing. Parishes or dioceses may seek to organize such efforts and end up giving rise to a broader healthcare ministry that cares for people according to the principles outlined in this book. Alternately, practice formation could be the initiative of a group of Catholic families who desire a different kind of medical care that respects the values they attempt to live out in the domestic churches of their households.

One foundation story behind an analogous educational enterprise that offers lessons for Benedict Medicine can be found in the origins of the Chesterton Schools Network. In 2007, concerned parents Dale Ahlquist and Tom Bengston in Minneapolis, Minnesota founded the first Chesterton school as a local initiative to offer an affordable, classical Catholic education option in their community.[3] When parents in other communities began to inquire how they could replicate the school's success and form their own local schools, a movement was born. Today, the Chesterton Schools Network has helped open sixty-nine schools across the United States and around the world, all modeled after the original joyfully Catholic Chesterton school in Minneapolis.[4]

The story of the Chesterton Schools Network invites several parallel observations between education and medical care. For one, both medicine and education are vital aspects of supporting the formation and flourishing of the human person—their human value goes well beyond grades, transcripts, or clinical assessments. How these enterprises engage in their work tells us about their meaning to those they serve. Medical services are not merely about preventing and treating disease, any more than education is merely about increasing pupils' standardized test scores or future economic attainment. How these entities carry out their functions is their statement of purpose.

---

3 For more information, see the Chesterton Schools Network website: https://chestertonschoolsnetwork.org/about.

4 Nora Kenney, "An Atmosphere of Joy," *City Journal*, February 14, 2024, https://www.city-journal.org/article/an-atmosphere-of-joy.

For clinicians seeking a greater congruence between their professional and their spiritual lives, the idea of transforming their practice of medicine can seem daunting. Particularly when one faces the uncertainty that drastic change can bring, the inertia of the status quo can seem like the safest option. Fear of the unknown is a potent tool of the adversary, and it has the capacity to neutralize our best intentions and prevent us from living the way the Lord calls us to live. For this reason, even the slightest initial step toward a more faithful practice draws us closer to the integrated Christian life.

For those medical professionals who prefer a more incremental approach to aligning practice and faith, the following questions provide a framework for how to begin.

- Do any areas of my current practice patterns or arrangement conflict with my Christian faith? When I started, did I consider these factors before choosing to enter this practice? What has changed both in the practice and in my life since that time?
- What external expectations of my current role work against the Catholic social teaching principles of human dignity, solidarity, subsidiarity, or stewardship?
- How might I alter my clinical practice patterns, my role within the institution, or the practice's workflow to align more closely with Christian principles?

The faithful who long for a medical practice that puts Christian principles front and center face a similar process of discernment. Most Americans search for a doctor by perusing the provider network offered by their insurance plan. Far from statements of mission or purpose, the common denominator among these practices is their agreement to accept the terms of the insurance company in exchange for a steady stream of patient referrals. Christians who wish to find a practice that adheres to Hippocratic principles and the concept of *imago Dei* may need to consider breaking out of the insurance herd mentality to find what they are seeking. Like anything worth pursuing, contributing to the growth and flourishing of an authentically Christian medical mission requires some sacrifice. Reflect on the following questions when considering how to proceed in this effort of seeking, developing, and supporting Benedict Medicine practices:

- Would I be willing to join with other like-minded people or families in my community to bring this type of medical care to my area, as did the families that developed the Chesterton Schools Network?
- Do I know a faithful medical practitioner who could use some encouragement and so be moved to participate in this process?

- ✠ Am I prepared to invest financially to support an independent Christian practice that honors Benedict Medicine principles?
- ✠ Do I pray regularly for Christian medical professionals, asking the Holy Spirit to guide their work?

Prayerful consideration of these questions is likely to help the discerning Christian to see how to support the flourishing of a faith-oriented medical practice that promotes the common good.

Business Structure

For many clinicians considering their own Benedict Medicine practices, the legal structure of the practice can present an agonizing decision. Many ask, "Should I form a corporation such as a limited liability company (LLC) or professional association (PA)? Or is it preferable to form the practice as a nonprofit organization?" Indeed, the business structure you choose will have implications for the way the practice operates, generates revenue, and addresses liability. Corporate structures such as LLCs and PAs allow the practice owner greater control in directing the operation and development of the practice. A 501(c)(3) nonprofit requires the oversight of a board of directors, but it can also apply for grant funding and appeal for tax-deductible donations.

This book is not intended to give advice on the pros and cons of each corporate structure option. To develop a practice aligned with the principles of Benedict Medicine, the mission is the most important aspect that defines its existence. Whether the mission is the product of a single physician's inspiration or the work of a group of parishioners looking to bring faith-informed practice to the parish community, being clear about the practice's goals and how they embody Catholic social teaching principles is the defining characteristic. This commitment should be prominently stated in the practice's mission statement, as well as promotional materials, practice website, and press releases. Remember the "why" behind your practice's formation, and proclaim it decisively. Your future patients will appreciate the boldness of your statement of faith.

Medical Practice as Community

Establishing a primary care practice grounded in Catholic social teaching requires integrating within the community. The practice must be visible to those who will most likely benefit from the care it provides, as well as people who may be attracted by an intriguing alternative to the status quo. A Benedict Medicine practice must be strong in adhering to the faith without being withdrawn or isolated. It cannot compromise with the surrounding culture on principles of truth, yet it must remain visible to all. It is a fortress for those practitioners and patients who yearn for medical care that sustains their desire to live faithful lives while serving as a beacon for others who may not have considered the importance of medical practice as an expression of Christian virtues. It decisively rejects the premise of the "neutral physician" (described in chapter 4), while still remaining open to care for people of all backgrounds, creeds, and walks of life who come for care.

Connecting with others who share this book's vision—whether in our practices, parishes, or dioceses—can instigate change and lead to the development of a decidedly Christian local medical response. Such medical practices can serve as a springboard for greater participation in living a spiritually and materially integrated life among all people who yearn for coherence between their Christian faith convictions and their daily lives. Amid the morally bankrupt social institutions that saturate the secular order, new structures that address our deeper commitments as Christians renew our hope and give us strength to continue to live virtuously in community. Far from promoting isolation and retreat, the strengthening of a visible Christian community is intended to invite others to experience the love of Christ through our ministry.

The necessary role of community in Benedict Medicine implies that the success of such a practice requires partnership, sacrifice, and investment at many levels. Far from depending wholly on individual physicians who take the risk of renouncing the financial security of conventional practice, this project depends on the collaboration of other organizations committed to the Christian ecosystem in the local community. Aside from the support of individual patients who entrust the Benedict Medicine practice with their health, other entities such as dioceses, parishes, religiously affiliated schools, homeschool groups, lay ministries, and small businesses are natural partners that advance their own missions through supporting independent Christian medical practices. By subsidizing their own employees' and families' enrollments in Benedict Medicine practices, and by sharing the mission and work of such healthcare ministries, partnering organizations share in practices' medical witness.

The Benedict Medicine Consortium

Christian community extends beyond geography for physicians and laypeople who are drawn to the idea of medical practice as mission. Called to form community and to support and encourage one another, a group of committed Catholic primary care physicians were motivated to come together and form the Benedict Medicine Consortium.[5] This

[5] Visit the Benedict Medicine Consortium online at https://benedictmedicine.org.

nascent voluntary organization exists to support a culture of Catholic primary care according to the principles outlined in this book. The consortium brings together faithful medical professionals who seek to live their faith through their practice of medicine. While many member physicians already live out the concept of medical localism or medical distributism, others are at different points on their pilgrimage toward a more faith-informed practice that is integrated with other facets of their lives. The aims of the consortium are to provide fellowship as well as practical encouragement to others walking this path of Christian discipleship through primary care medicine. As it grows, the consortium will increase its ability to serve as a resource for clinicians and laypeople alike who wish to build a culture of faithful primary care that can nurture and sustain local Christian communities.

Considering the state of the Church in our country today, faithful parallel institutions that serve Christian communities are needed now more than ever. As I said in the introduction, recent decades have brought a sharp decline in the role of faith, both in public life and in our secular institutions. At the same time, fewer and fewer people recognize the importance of faith in their daily lives and worldview. This hollowing-out of the Church was forecast by a young Fr. Joseph Ratzinger (later Pope Benedict XVI) in a 1969 address on German radio:

> From the crisis of today the Church of tomorrow will emerge—a Church that has lost much. She will become small and will have to start afresh more or less from the beginning. She will no longer be able to inhabit many of the edifices she built in prosperity. As the number of her adherents diminishes, so it will lose many of her social privileges. . . . The Church will be a more spiritual Church, not presuming upon a political mandate, flirting as little with the Left as with the Right. It will be hard going for the Church, for the process of crystallization and clarification will cost her much valuable energy. It will make her poor and cause her to become the Church of the meek.[6]

This prediction was a disturbingly accurate description of the state of the Church today, more than a half-century after his pronouncement. While quantitatively smaller, the Church today has in many ways become a more invigorated Church. Evidence exists in the development and growth of authentically Catholic colleges and universities across the

---

[6] Joseph Ratzinger, quoted and translated in Tod Worner, "When Father Joseph Ratzinger Predicted the Future of the Church," *Aleteia*, June 13, 2016, https://aleteia.org/2016/06/13/when-cardinal-joseph-ratzinger-predicted-the-future-of-the-church.

country, highlighted by those featured in the Cardinal Newman Society. The reemergence of classical Catholic K-12 education, such as the Chesterton Schools Network, also speaks to the zeal of young families who strive to live as domestic churches according to the faith.

Amid the secular pressures that intend to force compromise with the world, Christians must remain steadfast in the faith and learn from their two-thousand-year inheritance that withstood plagues and persecutions in faithful service to Christ Jesus. Constructing institutions that preserve the seeds of faith requires that we be radically countercultural in how we live. Among other activities, we must foster medical witness such as that envisioned by practices committed to the principles of Benedict Medicine outlined in this book. Such practices are instrumental in the formation of our families and communities, and they contribute to our efforts to live the Christian life. Like St. Benedict of Nursia, who exchanged the decadence of Rome in the early sixth century for a cave in Subiaco, Italy, today's Christians must not be afraid to publicly profess our faith through our actions. Far from shielding ourselves in retreat, we must respond to the culture's hostility by engaging with the world in the way our Lord instructs us: with faith, hope, and charity. Just as St. Benedict founded monasteries that preserved the Christian soul of Europe during the chaos and corruption after the fall of the Roman Empire and became the template for a new image of Christian community, today's Christians are enjoined to unite in faith as a civic act capable of transforming our own decaying civilization. May our prayer be that faithful medical ministries in the mold of Benedict Medicine continue to exemplify faith, hope, and charity as they grow in strength and number, and that the Christian communities who support them may be instruments of the Holy Spirit to restore medicine to its transcendent healing purpose.

About the Author

Dr. James O. Breen is a family physician and associate clinical professor in the Department of Family Medicine of Florida State University. He is the organizer of the Benedict Medicine Consortium, an association of Catholic clinicians working to integrate Catholic social teaching in primary care practice. His writing has appeared in such publications as *Crisis Magazine*, *The Catholic Thing*, and the *New England Journal of Medicine*, among others. He is a member of the Southwest Florida Guild of the Catholic Medical Association and has completed the Certification Program in Health Care Ethics of the National Catholic Bioethics Center. You can learn more about his work at JamesOBreen.com.

www.ingramcontent.com/pod-product-compliance
Lightning Source LLC
LaVergne TN
LVHW050937210926
848482LV00013B/651
9798218755423